Dosage Calculations Made Easy for Nursing Students

500+ Step-by-Step Practice Problems with Complete Solutions and Explanations

Stanley Lawrence Richardson

ISBN: 978-1-7642100-9-6
Isohan Publishing
First Edition: 2025

Table of Contents

Chapter 1: Mathematical Foundations for Medication Safety

Medication errors claim thousands of lives annually, and nearly half of these preventable tragedies stem from calculation mistakes. You stand at the threshold of a profession where mathematical precision saves lives—where the difference between 0.5 mg and 5 mg can mean the difference between healing and harm. This chapter builds the rock-solid mathematical foundation you need to calculate with confidence and protect every patient under your care.

Mathematics anxiety affects up to 80% of nursing students, yet mathematical competency remains non-negotiable in healthcare. The good news? Mathematical skills for medication administration follow predictable patterns that you can master through deliberate practice and proven techniques. Every calculation you perform connects directly to patient safety—making your mathematical journey both meaningful and manageable.

Understanding the Stakes

Patient safety depends on your ability to perform accurate calculations under pressure. Consider that medication administration represents one of the highest-risk activities in healthcare, with calculation errors accounting for 15-20% of all medication incidents. These statistics aren't meant to intimidate you—they highlight why mastering these skills matters so profoundly.

Your mathematical foundation needs to be automatic, reliable, and error-free. When a patient needs immediate medication, you won't have time to second-guess basic operations. You need mathematical fluency that allows you to focus on clinical judgment rather than computational mechanics.

Building Confidence Through Competence

Mathematical confidence grows through competence, not encouragement alone. You build competence by practicing until calculations become second nature—until your hands move automatically and your answers emerge correctly every time. This chapter provides that foundation through systematic skill building and extensive practice.

Diagnostic Pre-Assessment

Before building new skills, you need to identify your current mathematical strengths and areas needing attention. Complete these twenty problems to establish your baseline:

1. $0.25 + 0.125 =$ _____
2. $3/4 \div 1/8 =$ _____
3. 15% of 80 = _____
4. Round 2.847 to the nearest tenth = _____
5. $0.5 \times 250 =$ _____

Continue through all twenty problems, checking your work carefully. Don't worry if some answers feel uncertain—this assessment helps identify exactly where to focus your energy.

Fractions, Decimals, and Percentages Mastery

Healthcare calculations require fluent conversion between fractions, decimals, and percentages. You'll encounter medication strengths expressed as percentages (1% lidocaine), decimal dosages (0.25 mg digoxin), and fractional tablets (1/2 tablet of medication).

Fraction Fundamentals

Fractions represent parts of a whole, expressed as numerator over denominator. The numerator tells you how many parts you have; the denominator tells you how many parts make the whole. When calculating medication doses, fractions often represent portions of available tablets or liquid volumes.

For medication calculations, focus on these essential fraction operations:

Addition and Subtraction: Find common denominators before adding or subtracting fractions. If a patient receives 1/4 tablet in the morning and 1/2 tablet in the evening, convert to common denominators: 1/4 + 2/4 = 3/4 tablet total daily dose.

Multiplication: Multiply numerators together and denominators together. If 1/2 tablet contains 25 mg of medication, then 3/4 tablet contains: 3/4 × 25 mg = 75/4 mg = 18.75 mg.

Division: Multiply by the reciprocal (flip the second fraction). If you have 2/3 of a solution and need to divide it into 1/6 portions, calculate: 2/3 ÷ 1/6 = 2/3 × 6/1 = 12/3 = 4 portions.

Decimal Precision

Decimals provide precise measurements essential for medication safety. Understanding decimal place values prevents potentially fatal errors like confusing 0.5 mg with 5.0 mg.

Practice reading decimals aloud correctly:

- 0.125 = "zero point one two five" (never "point one twenty-five")
- 2.50 = "two point five zero" (trailing zeros matter in medication orders)
- 0.025 = "zero point zero two five"

Decimal Operations for Medications:

Addition and subtraction require aligning decimal points vertically. If a patient receives 1.25 mg in the morning and 0.75 mg in the evening, align decimals: $1.25 + 0.75 = 2.00$ mg total daily dose.

Multiplication involves counting total decimal places in both numbers, then placing the decimal point accordingly. Calculate 0.5 mg $\times$ 2.5 = 1.25 mg (one decimal place plus one decimal place equals two decimal places in the answer).

Division requires careful decimal placement. When dividing 12.5 mg by 2.5, set up the division and move decimal points as needed: $12.5 \div 2.5 = 5.0$ mg.

Percentage Applications

Percentages appear frequently in medication concentrations and solution strengths. A 1% solution contains 1 gram of medication per 100 mL of solution. Understanding percentage conversions helps you work with various medication formulations.

Convert percentages to decimals by moving the decimal point two places left:

- 5% = 0.05
- 0.25% = 0.0025
- 150% = 1.50

Rounding Rules for Medication Safety

Rounding rules in healthcare follow specific guidelines that prioritize patient safety over mathematical convenience. These rules help prevent both underdosing and overdosing while maintaining practical administration guidelines.

Standard Rounding Rules:

Round to the nearest tenth for most oral medications. If calculations yield 1.67 tablets, round to 1.7 tablets—but check if this makes clinical sense (can you actually give 1.7 tablets?).

Round to the nearest hundredth for injectable medications. Insulin doses calculated as 7.834 units round to 7.83 units, matching syringe measurement capabilities.

Round to the nearest whole number for capsules that cannot be split. You cannot give 2.3 capsules—round to 2 capsules and verify the dose remains safe and effective.

Special Considerations:

Pediatric medications often require more precise rounding due to smaller body weights and narrower therapeutic windows. Always verify that rounded doses fall within safe ranges for the patient's age and weight.

High-alert medications like insulin, heparin, and digoxin may require institution-specific rounding protocols. Learn these protocols during clinical orientation and follow them consistently.

Case Study Examples

Case Study 1: Medical-Surgical Unit

Maria Rodriguez, a 45-year-old post-operative patient, requires pain medication. The physician orders acetaminophen 650 mg every 6 hours. Available tablets contain 325 mg each.

Calculate the number of tablets needed: 650 mg ÷ 325 mg per tablet = 2 tablets per dose.

Verify the calculation: 2 tablets × 325 mg per tablet = 650 mg ✓

Check the daily total: 2 tablets × 4 doses per day = 8 tablets daily, providing 2,600 mg total daily dose—within safe limits for adults.

This straightforward calculation demonstrates basic division and verification techniques. Always check your work by multiplying back to the original dose.

Case Study 2: Pediatric Unit

Eight-year-old James Chen weighs 25 kg and needs amoxicillin. The standard pediatric dose is 20 mg/kg/day divided into three doses. Available suspension contains 125 mg per 5 mL.

First, calculate the total daily dose: 25 kg × 20 mg/kg/day = 500 mg/day.

Next, calculate the individual dose: 500 mg/day ÷ 3 doses/day = 166.67 mg per dose.

Round to 167 mg per dose for practical administration.

Calculate the volume needed: 167 mg ÷ 125 mg per 5 mL = 167 mg ÷ 25 mg/mL = 6.68 mL per dose.

Round to 6.7 mL per dose, which can be measured accurately with an oral syringe.

This calculation involves multiple steps: weight-based dosing, division into multiple daily doses, and volume calculation from concentration.

Case Study 3: Critical Care Unit

Robert Thompson, a 70-year-old patient with heart failure, needs digoxin loading dose. His weight is 80 kg, and the loading dose is 10 mcg/kg. Available vials contain 0.25 mg/mL (250 mcg/mL).

Calculate the required dose: 80 kg × 10 mcg/kg = 800 mcg total loading dose.

Convert to volume needed: 800 mcg ÷ 250 mcg/mL = 3.2 mL.

Verify by working backwards: 3.2 mL × 250 mcg/mL = 800 mcg ✓

This case demonstrates unit conversion (mg to mcg), weight-based dosing, and concentration calculations—all essential skills for critical care nursing.

Common Error Patterns and Prevention

Mathematical errors in healthcare follow predictable patterns. Recognizing these patterns helps you avoid them and double-check your work effectively.

Decimal Point Errors: The most dangerous errors involve misplaced decimal points. Always write leading zeros (0.5, not .5) and avoid unnecessary trailing zeros (5 mg, not 5.0 mg) unless required for clarity.

Unit Confusion: Keep track of units throughout calculations. If you start with mg, ensure your final answer includes appropriate units. Mixed units (mg, mcg, g) require careful conversion.

Proportion Setup Errors: When using ratios and proportions, maintain consistent unit relationships. If you write "mg : tablet" on one side, use "mg : tablet" on the other side.

Calculation Verification: Always verify calculations using a different method when possible. If you used division, check with multiplication. If you used one formula, verify with another approach.

Building Mathematical Confidence

Mathematical confidence builds through successful problem-solving experiences. Start with problems you can solve correctly, then gradually increase complexity. This approach builds competence and confidence simultaneously.

Practice daily, even if only for fifteen minutes. Consistent daily practice builds stronger skills than occasional long study sessions.

Use practice problems that mirror real clinical scenarios you'll encounter.

Work problems step-by-step, writing down each step clearly. This technique helps identify where errors occur and builds systematic problem-solving habits. Rushed calculations lead to careless errors.

Join study groups where you can explain your problem-solving process to classmates. Teaching others reinforces your own understanding and helps identify gaps in your knowledge.

Technology and Calculation Safety

While calculators provide computational support, you still need strong foundational skills to set up problems correctly and recognize unreasonable answers. A calculator cannot tell you that 50 mg is an unreasonable dose of digoxin for an adult.

Use technology wisely: employ calculators for complex computations, but verify that your setup and units make sense. Double-check critical calculations manually when time permits.

Learn your institution's policies about calculator use during competency testing. Some programs require manual calculations to ensure you can function when technology fails.

Wrapping Up: Your Mathematical Foundation

Mathematical competence provides the foundation for every medication calculation you'll perform throughout your nursing career. These basic skills—fraction operations, decimal precision, percentage calculations, and proper rounding—become the tools you use to protect patient safety every day.

Your mathematical journey doesn't end with this chapter; it begins here. Each subsequent chapter builds on these foundations, adding layers of complexity that mirror real clinical practice. Trust in your ability to master these skills through consistent practice and thoughtful application.

The mathematical precision you develop now will serve you throughout your career, whether you're calculating pediatric doses in a children's hospital or titrating vasoactive drips in an intensive care unit. Every calculation you perform connects directly to a human life—making your mathematical mastery both meaningful and essential.

Key Learning Points

- Mathematical precision in medication calculations directly impacts patient safety and clinical outcomes
- Fractions, decimals, and percentages require fluent conversion skills for accurate dose calculations
- Proper rounding techniques follow healthcare-specific guidelines that prioritize safety over mathematical convention
- Common error patterns can be prevented through systematic verification and careful unit tracking
- Mathematical confidence builds through competence gained via consistent practice and gradual skill progression

Chapter 2: Mastering Measurement Systems and Conversions

Healthcare operates in a world where precision measured in micrograms can determine life or death outcomes. You'll work with medications measured in milligrams, patient weights recorded in kilograms, and home care instructions given in teaspoons—often within the same shift. Mastering measurement system conversions transforms you from someone who struggles with numbers into a confident practitioner who moves seamlessly between systems.

The challenge isn't just learning conversion factors; it's developing the clinical judgment to know when conversions are necessary and the mathematical fluency to perform them accurately under pressure. This chapter provides the systematic approach you need to master conversions across all measurement systems used in healthcare.

The Three Systems You Must Know

Healthcare professionals work primarily with three measurement systems: metric (the international standard), household (what patients use at home), and apothecary (traditional pharmacy measurements still found in some contexts). Each system serves specific purposes, and you need fluency in all three.

The Metric System Foundation

The metric system provides the scientific basis for modern healthcare measurements. Built on powers of ten, it offers logical, consistent relationships between units that make calculations straightforward once you understand the patterns.

Understanding metric prefixes solves most conversion challenges. Each prefix represents a specific power of ten:

Kilo- means 1,000 (kilogram = 1,000 grams) Centi- means 0.01 (centimeter = 0.01 meter)
Milli- means 0.001 (milligram = 0.001 gram) Micro- means 0.000001 (microgram = 0.000001 gram)

These relationships create predictable conversion patterns. Moving from larger to smaller units requires multiplication; moving from smaller to larger units requires division. The number of decimal places moved corresponds to the power of ten difference between units.

Converting Within the Metric System

Weight conversions form the backbone of medication calculations. The basic progression runs: kilogram → gram → milligram → microgram. Each step represents a 1,000-fold change.

To convert kilograms to grams: multiply by 1,000 (move decimal three places right) 2.5 kg = 2,500 g

To convert grams to milligrams: multiply by 1,000 (move decimal three places right)
0.5 g = 500 mg

To convert milligrams to micrograms: multiply by 1,000 (move decimal three places right) 0.25 mg = 250 mcg

Reverse these operations when converting from smaller to larger units. Always move the decimal point—don't just add or remove zeros, which can lead to errors.

Volume measurements follow similar patterns. The basic progression runs: liter → milliliter. One liter equals 1,000 milliliters, making this conversion straightforward.

For practical nursing purposes, remember that 1 milliliter equals 1 cubic centimeter (cc), though "cc" is being phased out in many institutions due to potential confusion with other abbreviations.

Household Measurements for Home Care

Patients use household measurements at home, making these conversions essential for discharge planning and home care instructions. While less precise than metric measurements, household units provide familiar reference points for patients and families.

Essential household equivalents include:

- 1 tablespoon = 15 mL
- 1 teaspoon = 5 mL
- 1 fluid ounce = 30 mL
- 1 cup = 240 mL (8 fluid ounces)
- 1 pint = 480 mL (16 fluid ounces)
- 1 quart = 960 mL (32 fluid ounces)

Weight conversions between household and metric systems:

- 1 pound = 2.2 kilograms (or 1 kg = 2.2 pounds)
- 1 ounce = 30 grams

These conversions approximate rather than provide exact equivalents, but they offer sufficient precision for most clinical applications.

Apothecary System Remnants

The apothecary system appears less frequently in modern practice, but you'll still encounter it in some contexts. Key conversions include:

- 1 grain = 60 mg (approximately)
- 1 dram = 4 mL (approximately)

Some medications, particularly older formulations, may still list strengths in grains. Aspirin tablets, for example, might be labeled as 5 grains (approximately 325 mg).

Clinical Conversion Applications

Weight-Based Medication Dosing

Many medications require dosing based on patient weight, typically expressed as mg/kg or mcg/kg. These calculations demand accurate weight conversion between pounds and kilograms.

The conversion factor—1 kg = 2.2 pounds—appears simple, but applying it correctly requires attention to direction. Converting pounds to kilograms requires division by 2.2; converting kilograms to pounds requires multiplication by 2.2.

Practice with common weights helps build fluency:

- 150 pounds ÷ 2.2 = 68.2 kg
- 200 pounds ÷ 2.2 = 90.9 kg
- 25 kg × 2.2 = 55 pounds

Round weights to the nearest tenth of a kilogram for most calculations, unless your institution specifies different rounding protocols.

Solution Concentrations and Dilutions

Understanding concentration relationships helps you work with various medication formulations. Concentrations express the amount of active ingredient per unit of solution.

A 1% solution contains 1 gram of medication per 100 mL of solution, which equals 10 mg per mL. This relationship helps you convert between percentage concentrations and mg/mL concentrations commonly used in clinical practice.

Higher concentration solutions require smaller volumes to deliver the same dose. Lower concentration solutions require larger volumes. This relationship guides dilution calculations and helps you verify that calculated volumes make clinical sense.

Case Study Applications

Case Study 1: Emergency Department Weight Conversion

Sarah Mitchell arrives at the emergency department weighing 176 pounds. She needs medication dosed at 15 mg/kg for her condition.

First, convert her weight to kilograms: 176 pounds ÷ 2.2 = 80 kg

Calculate her medication dose: 80 kg × 15 mg/kg = 1,200 mg

Verify the conversion by working backwards: 80 kg × 2.2 = 176 pounds ✓

This case demonstrates the importance of accurate weight conversion for weight-based dosing. Small errors in weight conversion multiply when calculating medication doses.

Case Study 2: Pediatric Home Care Instructions

Three-year-old Emma Thompson needs acetaminophen at home. Her weight is 15 kg, and the dose is 15 mg/kg every 6 hours. The family has children's acetaminophen suspension containing 160 mg per 5 mL (1 teaspoon).

Calculate Emma's dose: 15 kg × 15 mg/kg = 225 mg per dose

Convert to household measurement: 225 mg ÷ 160 mg per 5 mL = 1.41 × 5 mL = 7.05 mL

Convert to teaspoons for family understanding: 7.05 mL ÷ 5 mL per teaspoon = 1.4 teaspoons

Round to 1.5 teaspoons (7.5 mL) for practical measurement at home.

Verify: 1.5 teaspoons × 5 mL per teaspoon = 7.5 mL 7.5 mL × 160 mg per 5 mL = 240 mg (close to prescribed 225 mg, within acceptable range)

This case shows how multiple conversion steps help families administer medications safely at home using familiar measurements.

Case Study 3: Critical Care Unit Concentration Conversion

Mr. Jackson requires a dopamine infusion. The pharmacy provides dopamine 400 mg in 250 mL of D5W, creating a concentration of 1.6 mg/mL. The physician orders 5 mcg/kg/min, and Mr. Jackson weighs 80 kg.

Calculate the hourly dose requirement: 5 mcg/kg/min × 80 kg = 400 mcg/min 400 mcg/min × 60 min/hour = 24,000 mcg/hour

Convert to mg/hour: 24,000 mcg/hour ÷ 1,000 = 24 mg/hour

Calculate infusion rate: 24 mg/hour ÷ 1.6 mg/mL = 15 mL/hour

This case demonstrates multiple conversions within a single calculation: weight-based dosing, time conversion (minutes to hours), unit conversion (mcg to mg), and concentration application.

Memory Aids and Clinical Tips

Visual Memory Aids

Create visual associations for common conversions. Picture a kilometer as ten football fields end-to-end (approximately 1,000 meters). Visualize a teaspoon as the small spoon from your kitchen flatware set—exactly 5 mL.

Use body references for quick estimations. An adult thumb from tip to first joint measures approximately 2.5 cm (1 inch). This provides a quick reference for wound measurements or medication preparations.

Fraction Simplification for Speed

Common conversion fractions can be simplified for faster mental calculation:

- 1 kg = 2.2 pounds can be approximated as 1 kg ≈ 2 pounds for quick estimates
- 1 fluid ounce = 30 mL simplifies many household conversions
- 1 teaspoon = 5 mL provides the foundation for most liquid medication instructions

These approximations work well for estimates and double-checking exact calculations, but use precise conversion factors for final dose calculations.

Unit Cancellation Method

Set up conversions so unwanted units cancel out, leaving only desired units. This method prevents errors and helps verify correct setup:

Converting 150 pounds to kg: 150 pounds × (1 kg/2.2 pounds) = 68.2 kg

The "pounds" units cancel, leaving "kg" as the final unit. This visual confirmation helps catch setup errors before they become calculation errors.

Technology Integration and Verification

Calculator Use and Verification

Calculators help with arithmetic but cannot substitute for understanding. You must still set up problems correctly and verify that answers make clinical sense.

When using calculators for conversions, double-check by working backwards or using a different method. If you calculate 50 kg from 110 pounds, verify: 50 kg × 2.2 = 110 pounds ✓

Mobile Apps and Reference Tools

Many healthcare institutions allow approved conversion apps during clinical practice. Learn to use these tools efficiently while maintaining your manual calculation skills for situations where technology isn't available.

Practice with both manual calculations and technology-assisted calculations to build confidence in multiple approaches. Technology should supplement, not replace, your fundamental conversion skills.

Common Conversion Errors and Prevention

Decimal Point Displacement

Moving decimal points incorrectly creates the most dangerous conversion errors. Always double-check decimal point placement by estimating whether your answer seems reasonable.

If converting 2.5 kg to grams yields 25 g, recognize immediately that this answer is too small. 2.5 kg should yield 2,500 g—a much larger number, not a smaller one.

Unit Mix-ups

Keep track of units throughout multi-step conversions. Write units with every number to maintain clarity about what you're calculating.

When converting between weight units (kg, g, mg, mcg), pay special attention to the magnitude of change. Each step represents a 1,000-fold difference—a significant change that should be reflected in your numerical answer.

Approximation vs. Precision

Know when approximations are acceptable and when precision is required. Quick estimates help verify calculations, but medication doses require precise conversions using exact conversion factors.

Use approximations for safety checks: "Does this answer make sense?" Use precise calculations for final dose determinations: "Exactly how much medication does this patient need?"

Key Reflections: Building Conversion Mastery

Measurement system mastery provides the foundation for accurate medication administration across all healthcare settings. Your ability to move fluidly between metric, household, and apothecary systems enables you to communicate effectively with patients, families, and healthcare teams while maintaining the precision necessary for safe patient care.

These conversion skills become automatic through practice and application. Start with the most common conversions you'll use daily: pounds to kilograms, teaspoons to milliliters, and within-metric-system conversions. Build confidence with these fundamentals before tackling more complex conversion challenges.

Each conversion you master expands your clinical capability. You become the nurse who can quickly convert a physician's metric order to household measurements for patient education, or accurately calculate weight-based doses for patients of all sizes. These skills distinguish competent practitioners from those who struggle with basic clinical calculations.

Key Learning Points

- Metric system mastery requires understanding prefix relationships and decimal point movement patterns
- Household measurement conversions enable effective patient education and home care planning
- Weight conversions between pounds and kilograms form the foundation for most weight-based medication dosing
- Multiple conversion steps often appear in single calculations, requiring systematic setup and verification
- Visual memory aids and approximation techniques provide quick verification tools for precise calculations

Chapter 3: The Three Essential Calculation Methods

Three calculation methods dominate medication mathematics: dimensional analysis, ratio-proportion, and the formula method. Each approach offers distinct advantages, and skilled practitioners choose methods based on problem complexity, personal preference, and verification needs. This chapter teaches all three methods, helping you develop the flexibility to solve any medication calculation with confidence.

Rather than advocating for one "best" method, successful nurses master multiple approaches. This redundancy provides backup methods for double-checking critical calculations and alternative approaches when one method feels unclear. Your goal is fluency across all three methods, creating a robust mathematical toolkit for clinical practice.

Dimensional Analysis: The Universal Method

Dimensional analysis (also called factor-label method or unit conversion method) provides the most systematic approach to medication calculations. This method treats every calculation as a series of unit conversions, making it particularly powerful for complex problems involving multiple steps.

The fundamental principle involves setting up conversion factors so unwanted units cancel out, leaving only desired units in the final answer. This visual confirmation helps prevent setup errors while providing built-in verification of correct problem structure.

Basic Dimensional Analysis Structure

Every dimensional analysis calculation follows the same pattern:

Starting Amount × (Conversion Factor 1) × (Conversion Factor 2) × ... = Final Answer

Each conversion factor is a fraction where the numerator and denominator represent equivalent amounts expressed in different units. The key skill involves arranging these fractions so units cancel appropriately.

Setting Up Conversion Factors

Conversion factors come from known equivalencies. If 1 tablet contains 250 mg of medication, you can write two conversion factors:

(1 tablet / 250 mg) or (250 mg / 1 tablet)

Choose the fraction that allows unwanted units to cancel. If you need to convert from mg to tablets, use the first fraction. If converting from tablets to mg, use the second fraction.

Step-by-Step Problem Solving

Consider this problem: A patient needs 500 mg of acetaminophen. Available tablets contain 250 mg each. How many tablets should you give?

Step 1: Identify what you're looking for (tablets) and what you're starting with (500 mg)

Step 2: Set up the starting amount: 500 mg

Step 3: Identify the conversion factor: 1 tablet = 250 mg

Step 4: Arrange the conversion factor to cancel mg and yield tablets: 500 mg × (1 tablet / 250 mg) = 2 tablets

Step 5: Verify unit cancellation: "mg" cancels out, leaving "tablets"

Step 6: Check your answer: 2 tablets × 250 mg/tablet = 500 mg ✓

Advanced Dimensional Analysis Applications

Complex problems require multiple conversion factors, but the principle remains identical. Each conversion factor eliminates one unwanted unit while introducing the desired unit.

Consider this multi-step problem: A 176-pound patient needs medication dosed at 0.5 mg/kg/day given every 12 hours. Available tablets contain 125 mg each. How many tablets per dose?

Step 1: Convert weight to kg: 176 pounds × (1 kg / 2.2 pounds) = 80 kg

Step 2: Calculate total daily dose: 80 kg × (0.5 mg / kg / day) = 40 mg/day

Step 3: Calculate dose per administration: 40 mg/day × (1 day / 2 doses) = 20 mg/dose

Step 4: Convert to tablets: 20 mg/dose × (1 tablet / 125 mg) = 0.16 tablets/dose

This problem demonstrates dimensional analysis power: each step flows logically from the previous step, with units providing continuous verification of correct setup.

Ratio-Proportion: The Traditional Method

Ratio-proportion creates equations based on equivalent relationships. This method works particularly well for straightforward medication calculations and provides excellent verification for other methods.

Understanding Proportions

A proportion states that two ratios are equal. In medication calculations, one ratio represents the known relationship (medication strength), and the other represents the unknown relationship (dose needed).

The basic format is: A : B = C : D (read as "A is to B as C is to D")

For medication calculations: Known mg : Known tablets = Desired mg : Unknown tablets

Cross-Multiplication Solution

Once you establish the proportion, solve by cross-multiplication: If A : B = C : D, then $A \times D = B \times C$

Step-by-Step Ratio-Proportion

Using the same problem from before: A patient needs 500 mg of acetaminophen. Available tablets contain 250 mg each.

Step 1: Set up the known ratio: 250 mg : 1 tablet

Step 2: Set up the unknown ratio: 500 mg : X tablets

Step 3: Create the proportion: 250 mg : 1 tablet = 500 mg : X tablets

Step 4: Cross-multiply: $250 \times X = 1 \times 500$

Step 5: Solve for X: $X = 500 \div 250 = 2$ tablets

Step 6: Verify: Does 250 mg : 1 tablet = 500 mg : 2 tablets? $250 \times 2 = 500 \times 1$? $500 = 500$ ✓

Fraction Form of Proportions

Some people find fraction format clearer than colon format:

Known mg / Known tablets = Desired mg / Unknown tablets

Using the same example: 250 mg / 1 tablet = 500 mg / X tablets

Cross-multiply: $250 \times X = 500 \times 1$ Solve: $X = 500 \div 250 = 2$ tablets

Choose the format that feels most intuitive to you, but be consistent within each calculation.

Formula Method: Direct Calculation

The formula method provides a direct approach using the equation:

Dose Desired / Dose on Hand × Vehicle = Amount to Give

This method works well for simple medication calculations where you know exactly what you want (dose desired) and what you have available (dose on hand and vehicle).

Understanding Formula Components

- **Dose Desired**: The amount of medication the patient needs
- **Dose on Hand**: The amount of medication in each available unit
- **Vehicle**: The form the medication comes in (tablets, mL, etc.)
- **Amount to Give**: Your final answer (number of tablets, mL to give, etc.)

Formula Method Application

Using our standard example: Patient needs 500 mg acetaminophen. Available tablets contain 250 mg each.

Dose Desired = 500 mg Dose on Hand = 250 mg
Vehicle = 1 tablet

Amount to Give = (500 mg / 250 mg) × 1 tablet = 2 tablets

Formula Method Limitations

The formula method works best for single-step calculations. Complex problems requiring multiple conversions often become cumbersome with this approach. Use the formula method for straightforward calculations, but consider dimensional analysis for multi-step problems.

Case Study Comparisons

Case Study 1: Pediatric Liquid Medication

Eight-year-old patient needs amoxicillin 250 mg. Available suspension contains 125 mg per 5 mL.

Dimensional Analysis Solution: 250 mg × (5 mL / 125 mg) = 10 mL

Ratio-Proportion Solution: 125 mg : 5 mL = 250 mg : X mL 125 × X = 5 × 250 X = 1,250 ÷ 125 = 10 mL

Formula Method Solution: (250 mg / 125 mg) × 5 mL = 2 × 5 mL = 10 mL

All three methods yield the same answer, demonstrating their equivalence for straightforward calculations.

Case Study 2: Complex Weight-Based Dosing

A 70 kg patient needs heparin at 18 units/kg/hour. Available concentration is 25,000 units in 250 mL.

Dimensional Analysis Solution: 70 kg × (18 units/kg/hour) × (250 mL / 25,000 units) = 12.6 mL/hour

This single setup handles weight-based dosing and concentration conversion simultaneously.

Ratio-Proportion Solution (requires multiple steps): Step 1: Calculate hourly dose: 70 kg × 18 units/kg/hour = 1,260 units/hour Step 2: Set up proportion: 25,000 units : 250 mL = 1,260 units : X mL Step 3: Cross-multiply and solve: X = (1,260 × 250) ÷ 25,000 = 12.6 mL/hour

Formula Method Solution (requires multiple steps): Step 1: Calculate hourly dose: 70 kg × 18 units/kg/hour = 1,260 units/hour Step 2: Apply formula: (1,260 units / 25,000 units) × 250 mL = 12.6 mL/hour

This case demonstrates dimensional analysis advantages for complex calculations: fewer steps and less opportunity for intermediate errors.

Case Study 3: Emergency Medication Calculation

A patient in cardiac arrest needs epinephrine 1 mg IV push. Available pre-filled syringes contain 1 mg in 10 mL (1:10,000 concentration).

All Methods Solution: This problem requires no calculation—the available dose matches the ordered dose exactly. Give the entire 10 mL syringe.

However, if only 1:1,000 concentration were available (1 mg in 1 mL), you would need:

Dimensional Analysis: 1 mg × (1 mL / 1 mg) = 1 mL

Ratio-Proportion: 1 mg : 1 mL = 1 mg : X mL, so X = 1 mL

Formula Method: (1 mg / 1 mg) × 1 mL = 1 mL

Method Selection Guidelines

Choose Dimensional Analysis When:

- Problems involve multiple conversion steps
- You need to convert between different unit systems
- The calculation involves complex relationships (weight-based dosing with time factors)
- You want built-in verification through unit cancellation

Choose Ratio-Proportion When:

- Problems involve simple, direct relationships
- You prefer traditional mathematical approaches
- You need to verify answers calculated by other methods
- Working with students who find proportions intuitive

Choose Formula Method When:

- Calculations are straightforward and single-step
- All units are already compatible (no conversions needed)
- You want quick solutions for routine calculations
- Working with familiar medication formulations

Error Prevention Across All Methods

Unit Tracking

Regardless of method, track units throughout calculations. Units provide immediate feedback about setup accuracy and help identify errors before they propagate through complex calculations.

Write units with every number, even intermediate calculations. This practice prevents unit-related errors and makes problem verification straightforward.

Reasonableness Checks

Always evaluate whether your answer makes clinical sense. If you calculate 15 tablets for a single dose, question your setup. Most single doses involve 1-3 tablets or 1-30 mL of liquid medication.

Use approximation to verify magnitude. If you expect approximately 2 tablets and calculate 0.2 tablets, check your decimal point placement or unit setup.

Multiple Method Verification

For critical calculations, solve using two different methods and compare answers. If methods disagree, review both setups to identify errors.

This verification approach works particularly well in clinical practice where you have time for double-checking but need confidence in your calculations.

Clinical Mastery: Choosing Your Mathematical Approach

Mathematical fluency across multiple calculation methods provides the flexibility and confidence you need for safe medication administration. Each method offers unique advantages, and your choice should match problem complexity and personal preference while maintaining accuracy and efficiency.

Dimensional analysis provides the most systematic approach for complex calculations, especially those involving multiple conversions or unfamiliar relationships. Its visual unit cancellation offers built-in verification that helps prevent common setup errors.

Ratio-proportion offers intuitive appeal for many nurses and works excellently for verification purposes. Its traditional format makes it easy to explain to students and colleagues.

The formula method provides quick solutions for routine calculations where relationships are straightforward and familiar.

Your professional goal involves developing fluency across all three methods, creating mathematical redundancy that ensures accurate calculations regardless of clinical circumstances or time pressures. This mathematical flexibility distinguishes confident practitioners from those who struggle when their preferred method doesn't fit specific problems.

Key Learning Points

- Dimensional analysis provides systematic approaches for complex calculations through unit cancellation verification
- Ratio-proportion creates intuitive solutions for direct relationship problems and excellent verification tools
- Formula methods offer efficient solutions for straightforward calculations with compatible units
- Method selection should match problem complexity while considering personal preference and verification needs
- Multiple method fluency provides mathematical flexibility and verification capabilities for critical calculations

Chapter 4: Oral Medication Calculations

Oral medications represent the most common route of drug administration, accounting for approximately 60% of all medication doses given in healthcare settings. Yet this familiarity can breed carelessness—leading to calculation errors that compromise patient safety. This chapter transforms you from someone who "estimates" oral doses into a practitioner who calculates with precision and confidence.

Oral medication calculations involve more than simple arithmetic. You must consider bioavailability differences between formulations, patient-specific factors affecting absorption, and practical limitations of tablet splitting or liquid measurement. These considerations make oral medication calculations both foundational and sophisticated.

Understanding Oral Medication Forms

Solid Dosage Forms

Tablets and capsules provide precise, stable dosing in convenient forms. However, each formulation presents unique calculation considerations that affect both accuracy and safety.

Regular tablets can often be split if scored, but splitting requires careful consideration. Half of a 10 mg tablet provides 5 mg, but splitting accuracy depends on tablet uniformity and your technique. Unscored tablets should never be split, as medication distribution may be uneven.

Enteric-coated tablets resist stomach acid to prevent gastric irritation or medication degradation. These tablets must never be crushed or split, limiting your dosing options to whole tablets only. If calculations yield fractional tablets of enteric-coated medications, you need alternative formulations or dosing adjustments.

Extended-release formulations provide controlled medication release over time. Like enteric-coated tablets, these cannot be altered. Crushing or splitting destroys the release mechanism, potentially creating dangerous dose dumping or therapeutic failure.

Capsules generally cannot be split, though some can be opened and contents mixed with food (verify with pharmacy first). Calculate capsule doses in whole numbers only, unless your institution has specific protocols for capsule manipulation.

Liquid Dosage Forms

Liquid medications offer precise dosing flexibility, especially for pediatric patients or adults with swallowing difficulties. However, liquid calculations require attention to concentration relationships and measurement accuracy.

Suspensions contain medication particles suspended in liquid. These require thorough mixing before measurement to ensure uniform concentration. Always shake suspensions well and measure immediately after mixing.

Solutions contain medication completely dissolved in liquid, providing consistent concentration throughout the bottle. While more stable than suspensions, solutions still require careful measurement for accuracy.

Elixirs and syrups contain medication in sweetened liquid bases. These formulations help mask unpleasant tastes but may contain alcohol or high sugar content—important considerations for certain patients.

Basic Tablet and Capsule Calculations

Single-Strength Calculations

Most tablet calculations involve straightforward proportion relationships. You know the tablet strength and need to determine how many tablets provide the prescribed dose.

The dimensional analysis setup follows this pattern: Prescribed dose × (1 tablet / tablet strength) = number of tablets

Consider this example: Prescribed dose is 400 mg. Available tablets contain 200 mg each. 400 mg × (1 tablet / 200 mg) = 2 tablets

Verification: 2 tablets × 200 mg/tablet = 400 mg ✓

Multiple-Strength Availability

Many medications come in multiple tablet strengths, requiring you to choose the most appropriate combination. Your goal involves minimizing the number of tablets while maintaining accuracy.

For example: Prescribed dose is 150 mg. Available tablets are 50 mg and 100 mg.

Option 1: Use 100 mg + 50 mg tablets = 2 tablets total Option 2: Use three 50 mg tablets = 3 tablets total

Option 1 provides the same dose with fewer tablets—generally preferable for patient compliance and swallowing ease.

Partial Tablet Calculations

When calculations yield partial tablets, consider practical and safety implications. Can the tablet be safely split? Does the partial amount make clinical sense?

Example: Prescribed dose is 375 mg. Available tablets contain 250 mg each. 375 mg × (1 tablet / 250 mg) = 1.5 tablets

This calculation suggests giving 1½ tablets. Verify that the 250 mg tablets are scored and can be split safely. If not, consult with the prescriber about dose adjustment or alternative formulations.

Liquid Medication Calculations

Concentration-Based Calculations

Liquid medications express concentration as amount of medication per volume of liquid (mg/mL, mg/5mL, etc.). Your calculation determines what volume provides the prescribed dose.

The dimensional analysis setup: Prescribed dose × (volume of liquid / amount of medication) = volume to give

Example: Prescribed dose is 300 mg. Available suspension contains 125 mg per 5 mL. 300 mg × (5 mL / 125 mg) = 12 mL

Verification: 12 mL × (125 mg / 5 mL) = 300 mg ✓

Pediatric Liquid Calculations

Pediatric patients often receive liquid medications, requiring precise volume measurements. Use oral syringes or calibrated measuring devices—never household spoons, which vary significantly in volume.

Consider this pediatric example: A 25 kg child needs acetaminophen at 15 mg/kg. Available suspension contains 160 mg per 5 mL.

Step 1: Calculate dose: 25 kg × 15 mg/kg = 375 mg Step 2: Calculate volume: 375 mg × (5 mL / 160 mg) = 11.7 mL

Round to 11.7 mL (measurable with oral syringe) or 12 mL if using less precise measuring device.

Home Care Conversion Considerations

Patients and families often need conversions to household measurements for home administration. While less precise than metric measurements, household conversions provide familiar references.

If the calculated dose is 7.5 mL, convert to household terms: 7.5 mL ÷ 5 mL per teaspoon = 1.5 teaspoons

Always provide both metric and household measurements when possible, emphasizing the importance of using proper measuring devices.

Case Study Applications

Case Study 1: Complex Diabetes Management

Margaret Foster, a 65-year-old woman with type 2 diabetes, needs metformin dose adjustment. Her physician prescribes metformin 850 mg twice daily. Available tablets include 500 mg, 750 mg, and 1000 mg strengths.

For the 850 mg dose, consider available options:

- 750 mg + 100 mg tablets: not available
- 500 mg + 350 mg: would require splitting 700 mg tablet (not available)
- 1000 mg tablet split: 1000 mg ÷ 2 = 500 mg (incorrect dose)

The calculation reveals that 850 mg tablets specifically are needed, or the prescription requires modification. This case demonstrates how availability constraints affect calculation approaches.

Contact the prescriber to discuss alternatives:

- Use 750 mg tablets if therapeutically acceptable
- Switch to extended-release formulation with different available strengths
- Compound 850 mg tablets through specialized pharmacy

This scenario emphasizes the importance of considering practical limitations alongside mathematical accuracy.

Case Study 2: Pediatric Antibiotic Therapy

Seven-year-old Michael Chen weighs 22 kg and needs amoxicillin for strep throat. The prescribed dose is 25 mg/kg twice daily. Available suspension contains 400 mg per 5 mL.

Calculate the individual dose: 22 kg × 25 mg/kg = 550 mg per dose

Calculate the volume needed: 550 mg × (5 mL / 400 mg) = 6.875 mL

Round to 6.9 mL for oral syringe measurement.

Verify the calculation: 6.9 mL × (400 mg / 5 mL) = 552 mg (acceptable variance from 550 mg)

Convert to household measurement for family reference: 6.9 mL ÷ 5 mL per teaspoon = 1.4 teaspoons (approximately 1⅜ teaspoons)

Provide clear instructions: "Give 6.9 mL (about 1⅜ teaspoons) by mouth twice daily using the oral syringe provided."

This case shows integration of weight-based dosing, liquid calculations, and family education considerations.

Case Study 3: Geriatric Polypharmacy

Robert Thompson, an 82-year-old man, takes multiple medications. His morning regimen includes:

- Lisinopril 10 mg (available as 5 mg tablets)
- Metoprolol 50 mg (available as 25 mg and 100 mg tablets)
- Furosemide 40 mg (available as 20 mg and 80 mg tablets)

Calculate tablets needed for each medication:

Lisinopril: 10 mg × (1 tablet / 5 mg) = 2 tablets of 5 mg strength

Metoprolol: 50 mg could be:

- Two 25 mg tablets = 2 tablets
- Half of one 100 mg tablet = 0.5 tablets (if scored and splittable)

Choose two 25 mg tablets to avoid splitting requirements.

Furosemide: 40 mg could be:

- Two 20 mg tablets = 2 tablets
- Half of one 80 mg tablet = 0.5 tablets (if scored and splittable)

Choose two 20 mg tablets for consistency with whole-tablet dosing.

Total morning tablets: 2 + 2 + 2 = 6 tablets

This case demonstrates how strength selection affects total pill burden—an important consideration for elderly patients who may struggle with medication adherence.

Special Considerations for Oral Medications

Tablet Splitting Safety and Accuracy

Only split tablets when absolutely necessary and clinically appropriate. Scored tablets indicate manufacturer intention for splitting, but unscored tablets may have uneven medication distribution.

When splitting is necessary:

- Use a tablet splitter device for consistency
- Split tablets immediately before administration
- Inspect split pieces for approximate equality
- Document when partial tablets are given

Never split:

- Enteric-coated tablets
- Extended-release formulations
- Capsules (unless specifically designed to open)
- Sublingual or buccal tablets

Crushing and Alternative Routes

Some patients cannot swallow whole tablets due to dysphagia, altered consciousness, or feeding tubes. Crushing tablets changes their characteristics and may affect absorption or cause safety issues.

Safe to crush (verify with pharmacy):

- Most immediate-release, uncoated tablets
- Some scored tablets designed for dose flexibility

Never crush:

- Enteric-coated formulations
- Extended-release or sustained-release tablets
- Sublingual tablets
- Hazardous medications (chemotherapy, hormones)

When crushing is necessary, use appropriate techniques:

- Use pill crusher or mortar and pestle
- Mix with small amount of appropriate liquid
- Administer immediately after crushing
- Clean equipment thoroughly between different medications

Bioavailability and Bioequivalence

Different formulations of the same medication may have different bioavailability—the amount and rate of drug absorption. This consideration particularly affects:

- Generic vs. brand name medications
- Different manufacturers of the same generic drug
- Immediate-release vs. extended-release formulations
- Tablet vs. liquid formulations

While most generic medications provide equivalent therapeutic effects, some patients may experience differences when switching formulations. Monitor patients carefully when changing between different manufacturers or formulations.

Measurement Tools and Accuracy

Oral Syringes for Liquid Medications

Oral syringes provide the most accurate measurement for liquid medications, especially volumes less than 10 mL. Key advantages include:

- Precise volume markings (often to 0.1 mL)
- No risk of confusion with injection syringes
- Easy administration directly into patient's mouth
- Reduced spillage compared to cups or spoons

Always use appropriately sized syringes:

- 1 mL syringes for doses less than 1 mL
- 3 mL syringes for doses 1-3 mL
- 5 mL syringes for doses 3-5 mL
- 10 mL syringes for doses 5-10 mL

Medicine Cups and Measuring Devices

Medicine cups work adequately for volumes greater than 5 mL but provide less precision than oral syringes. Read measurements at eye level with the cup on a flat surface to avoid parallax errors.

Graduated cylinders offer excellent accuracy for larger volumes but are typically used in pharmacy settings rather than patient care areas.

Household Measuring Device Limitations

Household spoons vary significantly in volume—from 3 mL to 7 mL for "teaspoons." This variation creates significant dosing errors when patients use kitchen utensils instead of medical measuring devices.

Always provide appropriate measuring devices with liquid medications and educate patients about measurement accuracy importance.

Therapeutic Reflection: Precision in Everyday Practice

Oral medication calculations form the foundation of safe medication administration across all healthcare settings. These calculations appear deceptively simple—often involving basic arithmetic—yet they require sophisticated clinical judgment about formulation appropriateness, measurement accuracy, and patient-specific considerations.

Your competence with oral medication calculations directly impacts patient safety and therapeutic outcomes. Errors in this fundamental area propagate throughout your practice, affecting everything from pain management to antibiotic effectiveness to chronic disease control.

The precision you develop with oral medication calculations builds confidence that carries into more complex areas of medication administration. Master these fundamentals thoroughly—they serve as the foundation for intravenous calculations, pediatric dosing, and critical care medication management.

Every tablet you calculate and every milliliter you measure represents a therapeutic intervention that can improve a patient's health or, if calculated incorrectly, cause harm. This responsibility makes your mathematical precision both meaningful and essential.

Key Learning Points

- Solid dosage forms require consideration of splitting safety and formulation characteristics that affect calculation options
- Liquid medication calculations demand attention to concentration relationships and precise volume measurement techniques
- Multiple tablet strengths allow optimization of pill burden while maintaining dosing accuracy
- Special populations require modified approaches that consider swallowing ability, compliance factors, and measurement capabilities
- Measurement tool selection significantly impacts dosing accuracy, with oral syringes providing superior precision for most liquid medications

Chapter 5: Injectable Medication Mastery

Injectable medications deliver therapeutic agents directly into body tissues, bypassing the unpredictable absorption characteristics of oral routes. This directness creates both opportunity and risk—opportunity for rapid, reliable therapeutic effects, and risk from immediate, irreversible drug delivery. Injectable medication calculations demand precision that exceeds oral medication requirements because errors cannot be recalled once the injection is given.

Your mastery of injectable calculations protects patients from the most dangerous medication errors while enabling you to provide life-saving therapies when oral routes fail or prove inadequate. This chapter develops the specialized skills needed for subcutaneous, intramuscular, and intravenous injection calculations.

Understanding Injectable Medication Characteristics

Bioavailability and Onset Differences

Injectable medications achieve 100% bioavailability—every microgram you inject reaches systemic circulation. This complete absorption contrasts sharply with oral medications, where bioavailability ranges from 30-90% depending on drug characteristics and patient factors.

Rapid onset characterizes most injectable medications. Subcutaneous injections typically begin working within 15-30 minutes, intramuscular injections within 10-20 minutes, and intravenous injections within seconds to minutes. This speed demands accuracy in your initial calculation because corrections may not be possible once therapeutic effects begin.

Concentration Variations and Standardization

Injectable medications come in numerous concentration variations, creating complexity in calculation and selection. Insulin, for example, comes in U-100 (100 units/mL), U-200 (200 units/mL), and U-500 (500 units/mL) concentrations. Each concentration requires different calculation approaches and syringe selections.

Heparin presents even greater concentration variety: 1,000 units/mL, 5,000 units/mL, 10,000 units/mL, and 20,000 units/mL for therapeutic use, plus 10 units/mL and 100 units/mL for flush solutions. This range necessitates careful attention to concentration identification and appropriate calculation methods.

Volume Limitations by Route

Each injection route has specific volume limitations that affect your calculation approach:

Subcutaneous injections typically accommodate 0.5-1.5 mL maximum, depending on injection site and patient factors. Volumes exceeding these limits require multiple injection sites or alternative routes.

Intramuscular injections allow larger volumes: 1-3 mL in adults (depending on muscle mass and site), 0.5-1 mL in children, and 0.5 mL maximum in infants. Deltoid muscle accommodates smaller volumes (1 mL maximum) compared to ventrogluteal or vastus lateralis sites.

Intravenous injections have no inherent volume limitations, but concentration and administration rate considerations affect calculation approaches.

Insulin Calculations: Precision for Survival

Understanding U-100 Insulin

U-100 insulin contains 100 units of insulin per milliliter—the most common concentration in clinical practice. This standardization simplifies calculations: units of insulin equal the volume in a U-100 insulin syringe.

If a patient needs 25 units of U-100 insulin, draw 25 units on a U-100 insulin syringe. The volume will be 0.25 mL, but you think in units, not milliliters, when using insulin syringes designed for U-100 insulin.

Insulin Syringe Selection

Choose insulin syringe size based on dose requirements:

- 30-unit syringes (0.3 mL): for doses up to 30 units
- 50-unit syringes (0.5 mL): for doses up to 50 units
- 100-unit syringes (1.0 mL): for doses up to 100 units

Using appropriately sized syringes improves measurement accuracy. A 10-unit dose measured in a 100-unit syringe provides less precision than the same dose measured in a 30-unit syringe.

Mixing Insulin Types

Some patients require combinations of rapid-acting and long-acting insulins. Mixing calculations involve adding individual doses while considering compatibility and stability.

Example: Patient needs 8 units rapid-acting insulin plus 20 units long-acting insulin. Total dose: 8 units + 20 units = 28 units

Draw the rapid-acting insulin first (clear before cloudy), then add the long-acting insulin to reach 28 total units on the syringe.

Alternative Insulin Concentrations

U-200 insulin contains 200 units per milliliter—twice the concentration of U-100. Calculations require careful attention to concentration differences.

If a patient needs 40 units of U-200 insulin: 40 units × (1 mL / 200 units) = 0.2 mL

This volume would be drawn in a standard syringe (not an insulin syringe), as insulin syringes are calibrated for U-100 concentration only.

U-500 insulin (500 units/mL) requires even more precise calculations and often specialized syringes or careful volume measurement in standard syringes.

Heparin Calculations: Anticoagulation Precision

Subcutaneous Heparin Dosing

Subcutaneous heparin prevents venous thromboembolism in hospitalized patients. Standard prophylactic doses range from 5,000-7,500 units every 8-12 hours, depending on patient risk factors and institutional protocols.

Common concentration for subcutaneous use: 5,000 units/mL in pre-filled syringes or vials.

Example calculation: Patient needs 5,000 units subcutaneous heparin. Available concentration is 5,000 units/mL. 5,000 units × (1 mL / 5,000 units) = 1 mL

This calculation yields exactly 1 mL—convenient for pre-filled syringes but requiring careful dose verification.

Weight-Based Heparin Protocols

Some institutions use weight-based subcutaneous heparin dosing for enhanced effectiveness. These protocols typically prescribe 50-75 units/kg every 8-12 hours.

Example: 80 kg patient receiving 60 units/kg every 12 hours. Dose calculation: 80 kg × 60 units/kg = 4,800 units

Volume calculation with 5,000 units/mL concentration: 4,800 units × (1 mL / 5,000 units) = 0.96 mL

Round to 1.0 mL for practical administration (within acceptable dosing range).

Heparin Flush Calculations

Heparin flushes maintain IV catheter patency. Typical concentrations include 10 units/mL and 100 units/mL, with volumes ranging from 1-3 mL depending on catheter type and institutional protocols.

Most heparin flushes come pre-prepared, but understanding calculations helps verify appropriateness and prepare flushes when pre-filled options aren't available.

Reconstitution Calculations: Powder to Solution

Understanding Reconstitution Principles

Many injectable medications come as stable powders requiring reconstitution with sterile diluent before administration. Reconstitution calculations determine final concentration based on powder volume and diluent added.

The key principle: final volume equals diluent volume plus powder displacement volume. Powder displacement volume varies by medication and must be considered for accurate concentration calculation.

Single-Strength Reconstitution

Most antibiotics offer single reconstitution options with predetermined final concentrations.

Example: Ceftriaxone 1 g vial for intramuscular injection

- Add 2.1 mL sterile water

- Final volume: 2.5 mL (includes 0.4 mL powder displacement)
- Final concentration: 1 g / 2.5 mL = 400 mg/mL

If the patient needs 500 mg: 500 mg × (1 mL / 400 mg) = 1.25 mL

Multiple-Strength Reconstitution Options

Some medications allow different final concentrations based on diluent volume added. These options provide flexibility for different dosing needs and volume limitations.

Example: Penicillin G potassium 1,000,000 units vial

- Add 4.6 mL diluent for 200,000 units/mL concentration
- Add 1.6 mL diluent for 500,000 units/mL concentration

Choose concentration based on dose requirements and volume limitations.

For 300,000 units dose: Using 200,000 units/mL: 300,000 units × (1 mL / 200,000 units) = 1.5 mL Using 500,000 units/mL: 300,000 units × (1 mL / 500,000 units) = 0.6 mL

Both options work, but the higher concentration provides smaller injection volume—often preferable for patient comfort.

Stability Considerations After Reconstitution

Reconstituted medications have limited stability. Most remain potent for 24-48 hours when refrigerated, but some require use within hours of reconstitution. Always check reconstitution instructions for specific stability information.

Label reconstituted medications with:

- Date and time of reconstitution
- Final concentration
- Expiration date and time

- Your initials

Syringe Selection and Reading

Syringe Size Selection

Choose syringe size based on volume to be administered, with considerations for measurement accuracy and injection comfort.

1 mL syringes: Use for volumes less than 1 mL when precision is critical. Graduated in 0.01 mL increments, these syringes provide excellent accuracy for small doses.

3 mL syringes: Appropriate for volumes 1-3 mL. Graduated in 0.1 mL increments, providing good accuracy for most injectable medications.

5 mL and 10 mL syringes: Use for larger volumes but with reduced measurement precision. Consider multiple smaller injections if volume exceeds site limitations.

Reading Syringe Measurements

Read syringe measurements at the leading edge of the plunger (closest to the needle). This technique provides consistent, accurate measurements regardless of syringe size or graduation marks.

For volumes between graduation marks, round to the nearest measurable increment. A 1 mL syringe can measure 0.37 mL accurately, but a 3 mL syringe should round this to 0.4 mL.

Needle Selection Considerations

Needle selection affects injection success and patient comfort but doesn't directly impact calculations. However, understanding needle characteristics helps you verify that calculated volumes are appropriate for selected injection routes.

Subcutaneous injections: 25-27 gauge, 3/8-5/8 inch needles
Intramuscular injections: 21-25 gauge, 1-1.5 inch needles (depending on patient size and injection site) Intravenous injections: 20-24 gauge for direct injection

Case Study Applications

Case Study 1: Diabetes Management in Hospital

Patricia Williams, a 58-year-old woman with type 1 diabetes, requires sliding scale insulin coverage. Her blood glucose is 280 mg/dL. The sliding scale protocol prescribes:

- Blood glucose 250-300 mg/dL: 6 units rapid-acting insulin subcutaneous
- Available insulin: U-100 rapid-acting in insulin pens

Since her blood glucose of 280 mg/dL falls in the 250-300 range, she needs 6 units of insulin.

Using U-100 insulin pen: Set dial to 6 units and inject subcutaneously.

No calculation required—insulin pens are pre-calibrated for U-100 concentration. However, always verify the insulin concentration matches the pen calibration before administration.

This case demonstrates how modern insulin delivery systems simplify calculations while maintaining the need for careful dose verification.

Case Study 2: Post-Operative Pain Management

Michael Rodriguez, a 45-year-old man, needs morphine for post-operative pain control. The physician orders morphine 8 mg intramuscular every 4 hours as needed. Available morphine comes in 10 mg/mL concentration.

Calculate the volume needed: 8 mg × (1 mL / 10 mg) = 0.8 mL

Verify: 0.8 mL × 10 mg/mL = 8 mg ✓

Use a 1 mL syringe for accurate measurement of 0.8 mL. Administer intramuscularly in appropriate site (ventrogluteal or vastus lateralis).

This case shows straightforward concentration calculations with considerations for syringe selection and injection site appropriateness.

Case Study 3: Antibiotic Therapy with Reconstitution

Seven-year-old Emma Chen needs ceftriaxone 750 mg intramuscular for severe pneumonia. Available: ceftriaxone 1 g vial requiring reconstitution.

Reconstitution instructions: Add 2.1 mL sterile water for injection to 1 g vial. Final volume: 2.5 mL. Final concentration: 400 mg/mL.

Calculate volume needed for 750 mg dose: 750 mg × (1 mL / 400 mg) = 1.875 mL

Round to 1.9 mL for practical measurement with 3 mL syringe.

Verify: 1.9 mL × 400 mg/mL = 760 mg (acceptable variance from 750 mg)

This case integrates reconstitution calculations with pediatric dosing considerations and practical measurement limitations.

High-Alert Medication Protocols

Double-Check Requirements

High-alert medications like insulin, heparin, and chemotherapy require independent double-checks by two qualified staff members. This verification process includes:

- Calculation verification
- Concentration confirmation

- Dose appropriateness review
- Administration route verification

Both practitioners must independently perform calculations and compare results before administration.

Standardized Concentrations

Many institutions use standardized concentrations for high-alert medications to reduce calculation complexity and error risk. Learn your institution's standard concentrations and use them consistently.

Common standardizations include:

- Heparin: 5,000 units/mL for subcutaneous use
- Insulin: U-100 concentration for routine use
- Morphine: 10 mg/mL for intramuscular injection

Error Prevention Strategies

Use leading zeros for decimal doses (0.5 mg, not .5 mg) and avoid trailing zeros (5 mg, not 5.0 mg) unless required for clarity.

Store different concentrations of the same medication in separate locations to prevent selection errors.

Verify calculations using different methods: if you used dimensional analysis, verify with ratio-proportion or formula method.

Professional Foundation: Building Injectable Expertise

Injectable medication calculations require heightened precision because of their immediate, irreversible effects and potential for serious harm if calculated incorrectly. Your competence with these calculations enables you to provide life-saving therapies while protecting patients from medication errors that could cause permanent injury or death.

The mathematical principles remain consistent across all injectable routes—dimensional analysis, ratio-proportion, and formula methods all apply equally. However, the clinical considerations multiply: route-specific volume limitations, concentration variations, reconstitution requirements, and high-alert medication protocols all demand your attention alongside mathematical accuracy.

Your professional growth involves building confidence with these complex calculations while maintaining the healthy respect for their potential consequences that keeps patients safe. Each injection you calculate and administer represents a therapeutic intervention that requires both mathematical precision and clinical judgment.

The expertise you develop with injectable medications becomes foundational for advanced practice areas like critical care, where titrated drips and emergency medications require split-second calculation accuracy under extreme pressure.

Key Learning Points

- Injectable medications achieve complete bioavailability, making calculation accuracy more critical than with oral routes
- Insulin calculations require attention to concentration differences and appropriate syringe selection for measurement accuracy
- Heparin calculations involve multiple concentration options and weight-based dosing protocols that demand careful setup
- Reconstitution calculations must account for powder displacement volume to determine accurate final concentrations
- High-alert medication protocols require independent verification and standardized approaches to prevent calculation errors

Chapter 6: Intravenous Calculations and Flow Rates

Intravenous therapy represents the most direct and rapidly acting route of medication administration, delivering therapeutic agents directly into the circulatory system where they achieve immediate distribution throughout the body. This immediacy creates both therapeutic opportunity and profound responsibility—you can save lives with precisely calculated IV medications, or cause irreversible harm through calculation errors that cannot be retrieved once the medication enters the bloodstream

Understanding IV Flow Rate Fundamentals

Infusion Pump Programming Basics

Most modern healthcare facilities rely on infusion pumps that calculate in milliliters per hour (mL/hr). These devices provide precise, consistent delivery rates while offering safety features like occlusion detection and dose limits. Your role involves calculating the appropriate mL/hr rate and programming it correctly into the pump system.

The basic relationship for pump calculations follows this pattern:
Total volume to infuse ÷ Time in hours = mL/hr rate

This formula applies whether you're infusing maintenance fluids, intermittent medications, or continuous drip medications. Understanding this relationship helps you verify pump programming and troubleshoot delivery issues.

Gravity Infusion Calculations

Some clinical situations require gravity infusions without pump assistance. These calculations involve drops per minute based on the IV tubing's drop factor—the number of drops that equal one milliliter.

51

Standard drop factors include:

- Macrodrip tubing: 10, 15, or 20 drops/mL (varies by manufacturer)
- Microdrip tubing: 60 drops/mL (universal standard)

The gravity infusion formula: (Total volume × Drop factor) ÷ Time in minutes = Drops per minute

Microdrip tubing simplifies calculations because 60 drops/mL means that mL/hr equals drops/minute when using 60-drop tubing.

Time and Volume Relationships

IV calculations often require determining how long an infusion will run or what volume will infuse over a specific time period. These relationships help you plan patient care and coordinate medication timing.

Time calculation: Total volume ÷ mL/hr rate = Hours to complete
Volume calculation: mL/hr rate × Hours = Total volume infused

Basic IV Rate Calculations

Maintenance Fluid Calculations

Maintenance fluids replace normal physiologic losses and maintain homeostasis. Adult maintenance typically ranges from 1,500-3,000 mL per day, depending on patient size, clinical condition, and losses from fever, respiratory conditions, or other factors.

Example: A patient needs 2,400 mL of normal saline over 24 hours. 2,400 mL ÷ 24 hours = 100 mL/hr

Verify: 100 mL/hr × 24 hours = 2,400 mL ✓

Intermittent Medication Infusions

Many IV medications infuse over specific time periods to maintain therapeutic levels while minimizing adverse effects. Antibiotic infusions commonly run over 30-60 minutes to reduce the risk of phlebitis and maintain effective blood levels.

Example: Vancomycin 1 g in 250 mL normal saline to infuse over 60 minutes. 250 mL ÷ 1 hour = 250 mL/hr

If using gravity infusion with 15-drop tubing: (250 mL × 15 drops/mL) ÷ 60 minutes = 62.5 drops/minute

Round to 63 drops/minute for practical counting.

Bolus and Loading Dose Calculations

Some medications require rapid administration for immediate therapeutic effect. These bolus calculations determine infusion rates for specific volumes over short time periods.

Example: Normal saline 500 mL bolus over 30 minutes for volume resuscitation. 500 mL ÷ 0.5 hours = 1,000 mL/hr

This high rate requires pump capability verification—ensure the pump can deliver 1,000 mL/hr and that IV access can accommodate this flow rate.

Drop Factor Applications

Macrodrip Calculations

Macrodrip tubing works well for routine fluid administration and intermittent medications. The larger drop size provides easier visual monitoring but requires more complex calculations than microdrip tubing.

Example: 1,000 mL lactated Ringer's solution over 8 hours using 10-drop tubing.

Step 1: Calculate mL/hr: 1,000 mL ÷ 8 hours = 125 mL/hr Step 2: Calculate drops/minute: (125 mL/hr × 10 drops/mL) ÷ 60 minutes/hr = 20.8 drops/minute

Round to 21 drops/minute for practical administration.

Microdrip Advantages

Microdrip tubing offers calculation simplicity because mL/hr equals drops/minute when using 60-drop factors. This relationship makes verification straightforward and reduces calculation complexity.

Example: Medication infusion at 50 mL/hr using microdrip tubing. 50 mL/hr = 50 drops/minute (no calculation required)

Use microdrip tubing for:

- Pediatric patients requiring precise, small volume control
- Medications requiring exact flow rates
- Situations where calculation simplicity improves safety

Visual Drop Counting Techniques

When monitoring gravity infusions, count drops over 15-30 seconds and multiply to determine per-minute rates. Longer counting periods provide more accurate averages but may be impractical in busy clinical settings.

15-second count × 4 = drops/minute 30-second count × 2 = drops/minute

Adjust flow rates gradually—small changes in roller clamp position create significant flow rate changes.

Time and Volume Calculations

Infusion Completion Timing

Calculating when infusions will complete helps coordinate patient care and medication scheduling. This planning prevents delays in subsequent treatments and ensures appropriate monitoring.

Example: 500 mL antibiotic infusion starts at 0800 and runs at 100 mL/hr. Completion time: 500 mL ÷ 100 mL/hr = 5 hours Infusion completes at: 0800 + 5 hours = 1300 (1:00 PM)

Volume Remaining Calculations

During infusions, you may need to calculate remaining volume and time to help with care planning and troubleshooting.

Example: 1,000 mL infusion started at 0600 at 125 mL/hr. At 1000, how much volume remains?

Time elapsed: 1000 - 0600 = 4 hours Volume infused: 125 mL/hr × 4 hours = 500 mL Volume remaining: 1,000 mL - 500 mL = 500 mL

Time remaining: 500 mL ÷ 125 mL/hr = 4 hours Completion time: 1000 + 4 hours = 1400 (2:00 PM)

Rate Adjustment Calculations

Sometimes infusions fall behind or get ahead of schedule, requiring rate adjustments to complete on time. These calculations determine new rates needed to finish infusions within prescribed timeframes.

Example: 1,000 mL infusion should complete in 8 hours but only 600 mL has infused after 6 hours. Calculate the new rate to finish on time.

Volume remaining: 1,000 mL - 600 mL = 400 mL Time remaining: 8 hours - 6 hours = 2 hours New rate needed: 400 mL ÷ 2 hours = 200 mL/hr

Verify this rate adjustment is safe and within medication guidelines before implementing.

Case Study Applications

Case Study 1: Post-Operative Fluid Management

Jennifer Martinez, a 35-year-old woman, returns from surgery needing fluid replacement. The physician orders 1,500 mL lactated Ringer's solution over 12 hours, followed by maintenance fluids at 100 mL/hr.

Calculate the initial infusion rate: 1,500 mL ÷ 12 hours = 125 mL/hr

Program the infusion pump for 125 mL/hr with a total volume of 1,500 mL. The pump will automatically alarm when this volume completes, prompting the rate change to 100 mL/hr for maintenance.

Timeline planning:

- Surgery completion: 1400
- Initial infusion completion: 1400 + 12 hours = 0200 (next day)
- Maintenance fluids begin: 0200

This case demonstrates basic pump programming with planned rate changes and timeline coordination.

Case Study 2: Pediatric Antibiotic Administration

Four-year-old David Kim weighs 18 kg and needs cefazolin 25 mg/kg every 8 hours. Each dose should infuse over 30 minutes. Available concentration: cefazolin 100 mg/mL.

Calculate the dose: 18 kg × 25 mg/kg = 450 mg per dose

Calculate volume needed: 450 mg × (1 mL / 100 mg) = 4.5 mL

This small volume requires dilution for safe 30-minute infusion. Mix with 20 mL normal saline for total volume of 24.5 mL.

Calculate infusion rate: 24.5 mL ÷ 0.5 hours = 49 mL/hr

Use microdrip tubing if pump unavailable: 49 mL/hr = 49 drops/minute

This case shows integration of weight-based dosing, volume calculations, dilution considerations, and infusion rate determination for pediatric patients.

Case Study 3: Critical Care Fluid Resuscitation

Robert Thompson, a 70-year-old man with sepsis, needs aggressive fluid resuscitation. The physician orders normal saline 30 mL/kg over 3 hours. Mr. Thompson weighs 80 kg.

Calculate total volume needed: 80 kg × 30 mL/kg = 2,400 mL

Calculate infusion rate: 2,400 mL ÷ 3 hours = 800 mL/hr

This high flow rate requires:

- Large-bore IV access (18-gauge or larger)
- Pump capable of high flow rates
- Frequent monitoring for signs of fluid overload
- Accurate intake/output documentation

Monitor for complications like pulmonary edema or heart failure exacerbation during rapid fluid administration.

Multiple IV Lines and Compatibility

Simultaneous Infusion Management

Many patients receive multiple IV infusions simultaneously through different lumens of central venous catheters or separate peripheral IVs. Each infusion requires independent calculation and monitoring.

Example: Patient with triple-lumen central line receiving:

- Lumen 1: Normal saline maintenance at 75 mL/hr

- Lumen 2: Vancomycin 1 g in 250 mL over 2 hours
- Lumen 3: Norepinephrine drip at 8 mL/hr

Calculate vancomycin rate: 250 mL ÷ 2 hours = 125 mL/hr

Total hourly fluid intake: 75 + 125 + 8 = 208 mL/hr

This calculation helps monitor total fluid balance and prevent fluid overload.

Medication Compatibility Considerations

Some medications cannot infuse through the same lumen due to chemical incompatibilities that cause precipitation or inactivation. These compatibility restrictions affect your infusion planning and timing.

Common incompatibilities include:

- Phenytoin with dextrose-containing solutions
- Calcium-containing solutions with phosphate-containing solutions
- Many antibiotics with each other

When compatibility data is unclear, flush lines with normal saline between different medications or use separate lumens when available.

Y-Site Administration Calculations

Y-site administration allows medication delivery through existing IV lines without interrupting primary infusions. These calculations determine appropriate flow rates for both primary and secondary infusions.

Example: Primary infusion of normal saline at 100 mL/hr with secondary antibiotic infusion of 50 mL over 30 minutes.

Secondary rate: 50 mL ÷ 0.5 hours = 100 mL/hr

During the 30-minute antibiotic infusion, the patient receives both fluids simultaneously. After antibiotic completion, primary infusion resumes at original rate.

Emergency IV Calculations

Rapid Sequence Medications

Emergency situations often require multiple medications in rapid succession. Each calculation must be accurate despite time pressure and stressful conditions.

Example: Cardiac arrest medications for 70 kg patient:

- Epinephrine 1 mg IV push (available 1:10,000 = 0.1 mg/mL): Give 10 mL
- Amiodarone 300 mg IV (available 50 mg/mL): Give 6 mL
- Sodium bicarbonate 1 mEq/kg (available 1 mEq/mL): Give 70 mL

These calculations require immediate accuracy without time for multiple verification methods. Practice emergency calculations regularly to build automaticity.

Vasoactive Medication Initiation

Critical care vasoactive medications often start with loading doses followed by continuous infusions. These calculations integrate bolus and drip rate determinations.

Example: Esmolol for hypertensive emergency

- Loading dose: 500 mcg/kg over 1 minute
- Maintenance infusion: 50 mcg/kg/minute

For 80 kg patient: Loading dose: 80 kg × 500 mcg/kg = 40,000 mcg = 40 mg Available concentration: 10 mg/mL Loading volume: 40 mg ÷ 10 mg/mL = 4 mL over 1 minute

Maintenance calculation (see Chapter 8 for detailed drip calculations): 80 kg × 50 mcg/kg/minute = 4,000 mcg/minute = 4 mg/minute

Technology Integration and Safety

Smart Pump Programming

Modern smart pumps contain drug libraries with pre-programmed dose limits and rate restrictions. These systems provide additional safety layers but require accurate programming to function effectively.

Key programming steps:

1. Select correct medication from pump library
2. Enter patient weight when required
3. Input calculated dose or rate
4. Verify pump calculations match your manual calculations
5. Review and confirm all pump settings before starting

Smart pumps alert you to potentially dangerous doses or rates, but they cannot substitute for accurate initial calculations.

Bar Code Medication Administration

BCMA systems verify medication identity but do not verify calculation accuracy. You remain responsible for ensuring calculated doses and rates are correct before scanning and administering medications.

Always verify that:

- Scanned medication matches calculated requirements
- Concentration on medication label matches your calculation assumptions
- Pump programming reflects your calculated rate

Electronic Documentation Integration

Many IV pumps integrate with electronic health records, automatically documenting infusion rates and volumes. Verify that automated documentation accurately reflects actual administration and make corrections when necessary.

Monitor pump accuracy by comparing documented volumes with actual fluid levels in IV bags or bottles. Significant discrepancies may indicate pump malfunctions requiring immediate attention.

Essential Mastery: IV Calculation Proficiency

Intravenous calculation mastery represents a cornerstone of safe nursing practice across all healthcare environments. Your ability to accurately calculate flow rates, determine infusion times, and manage multiple concurrent infusions directly impacts patient safety and therapeutic outcomes in ways that extend far beyond simple mathematical computation.

The immediacy and irreversibility of IV medications demand calculation accuracy that exceeds requirements for other administration routes. Each milliliter per hour you program into an infusion pump, each drop per minute you count in a gravity infusion, represents a clinical decision that affects patient physiology within minutes of implementation.

Your professional competence with IV calculations enables you to function confidently in emergency situations where split-second decisions save lives, manage complex critical care patients requiring multiple vasoactive drips, and provide safe, effective medication administration across diverse patient populations and clinical settings.

These skills form the foundation for advanced practice areas like critical care nursing, emergency medicine, and surgical services where IV medication expertise distinguishes competent practitioners from those who struggle with fundamental patient care responsibilities.

Key Learning Points

- Infusion pump calculations require accurate mL/hr determinations based on volume and time relationships
- Gravity infusion calculations depend on drop factor understanding and accurate drops-per-minute counting techniques
- Time and volume calculations enable effective care planning and infusion monitoring throughout administration periods
- Multiple IV line management requires systematic approaches to flow rate calculations and compatibility considerations
- Emergency IV calculations demand automaticity and accuracy under extreme time pressure and stressful clinical conditions

Chapter 7: Pediatric and Weight-Based Dosing

Pediatric medication calculations represent the highest-stakes mathematical challenges in healthcare. Children are not simply small adults—their physiologic differences create unique vulnerabilities that make calculation errors particularly dangerous. Pediatric patients have smaller margin for error, limited ability to communicate adverse effects, and rapidly changing body compositions that affect medication distribution and elimination.

Weight-based dosing extends beyond pediatrics to include many adult medications, but the principles reach their most critical application in children where therapeutic windows are narrow and overdose risks are amplified. This chapter develops the specialized skills needed to calculate medications safely across all age groups while paying special attention to pediatric considerations.

Understanding Pediatric Physiology and Dosing Principles

Age-Related Pharmacokinetic Changes

Pediatric medication metabolism differs significantly from adult patterns. Neonates and infants have immature liver enzymes and kidney function, leading to prolonged medication effects and potential toxicity from standard doses. School-age children often metabolize medications faster than adults, sometimes requiring higher per-kilogram doses to achieve therapeutic effects.

These physiologic differences explain why pediatric dosing relies heavily on weight-based calculations rather than standard doses. A medication dose that works safely for a 70 kg adult could be lethal for a 7 kg infant, even when adjusted proportionally for weight differences.

Body Surface Area Considerations

Some pediatric medications, particularly chemotherapy and certain high-risk drugs, use body surface area (BSA) calculations instead of simple weight-based dosing. BSA calculations account for the relationship between body size and metabolic rate more accurately than weight alone.

The most common BSA formula uses height and weight: BSA (m²) = $\sqrt{[(\text{Height in cm} \times \text{Weight in kg}) \div 3{,}600]}$

Alternatively, use BSA nomograms that provide visual lookup tools for common height and weight combinations.

Therapeutic Window Considerations

Pediatric therapeutic windows—the difference between effective and toxic doses—are often narrower than adult windows. This narrow margin demands exceptional calculation accuracy because small errors can push doses into either ineffective or dangerous ranges.

For example, digoxin therapeutic levels in children range from 1.0-2.0 ng/mL, with toxicity occurring above 2.5 ng/mL. This narrow window leaves little room for dosing errors that could cause heart rhythm disturbances or other serious complications.

Weight Conversion Mastery

Pound to Kilogram Conversion Accuracy

Accurate weight conversion forms the foundation of all weight-based calculations. The conversion factor—1 kg = 2.2 pounds—must be applied correctly and consistently.

Converting pounds to kilograms: Weight in pounds ÷ 2.2 = Weight in kg Converting kilograms to pounds: Weight in kg × 2.2 = Weight in pounds

Practice with common pediatric weights builds fluency:

- 22 pounds ÷ 2.2 = 10 kg
- 44 pounds ÷ 2.2 = 20 kg
- 66 pounds ÷ 2.2 = 30 kg

Round weights to the nearest tenth of a kilogram for most calculations, unless institutional protocols specify different precision requirements.

Growth Chart Integration

Pediatric weights change rapidly, especially during infancy. Always verify that weights are current and age-appropriate using growth charts. A weight that seems appropriate for a stated age should match expected percentiles on standardized growth curves.

Weights that fall far outside expected ranges warrant verification:

- Measure weight again
- Check for documentation errors
- Consider medical conditions affecting growth
- Consult with physicians about dose appropriateness

Weight Estimation Methods

Emergency situations sometimes require medication calculation before accurate weights can be obtained. Several estimation methods help provide reasonable approximations:

Broselow tape: Color-coded tape that correlates length with estimated weight for emergency situations. Provides reasonable estimates for children up to approximately 35 kg.

Age-based estimates:

- Age 1-10 years: Weight (kg) = (Age × 2) + 8
- Age 11-18 years: Use standard growth charts or direct measurement

These estimates should only be used when accurate weights cannot be obtained and immediate medication administration is necessary.

mg/kg and mcg/kg Calculations

Understanding Dose Expression Variations

Pediatric medications express doses in multiple formats that require careful interpretation:

- mg/kg/day: Total daily dose divided into appropriate number of individual doses
- mg/kg/dose: Amount given per individual administration
- mg/kg/hour: Continuous infusion rate calculation
- mcg/kg/minute: High-precision dosing for critical care medications

Always verify which format the prescription uses to avoid calculation errors that could result in significant over- or underdosing.

Daily Dose vs. Individual Dose Calculations

Many pediatric antibiotics prescribe total daily doses that divide into 2-4 individual administrations. Understanding this distinction prevents dangerous calculation errors.

Example: Amoxicillin 40 mg/kg/day divided every 8 hours for 20 kg child

Step 1: Calculate total daily dose: 20 kg × 40 mg/kg/day = 800 mg/day Step 2: Determine dosing frequency: Every 8 hours = 3 doses per day Step 3: Calculate individual dose: 800 mg/day ÷ 3 doses/day = 267 mg per dose

Continuous Infusion Calculations

Critical care pediatric medications often require continuous infusions with rates expressed as mcg/kg/minute or mg/kg/hour. These calculations integrate weight-based dosing with time factors.

Example: Dopamine 5 mcg/kg/minute for 25 kg child

Step 1: Calculate per-minute dose: 25 kg × 5 mcg/kg/minute = 125 mcg/minute Step 2: Convert to hourly dose: 125 mcg/minute × 60 minutes/hour = 7,500 mcg/hour Step 3: Convert to mg/hour: 7,500 mcg/hour ÷ 1,000 = 7.5 mg/hour

This hourly dose calculation enables infusion pump programming and medication preparation.

Safe Dose Range Verification

Understanding Pediatric Reference Ranges

Pediatric medication references provide safe dose ranges rather than single recommended doses. These ranges account for variation in patient conditions, severity of illness, and individual response patterns.

Example reference: Acetaminophen 10-15 mg/kg/dose every 4-6 hours (maximum 75 mg/kg/day)

For 15 kg child:

- Minimum safe dose: 15 kg × 10 mg/kg = 150 mg per dose
- Maximum safe dose: 15 kg × 15 mg/kg = 225 mg per dose
- Maximum daily dose: 15 kg × 75 mg/kg = 1,125 mg per day

Any calculated dose outside these ranges requires physician consultation before administration.

Dose Escalation and Frequency Considerations

Some pediatric medications allow dose increases based on patient response, but these escalations must remain within published safety limits. Track cumulative daily doses to ensure maximum limits are not exceeded.

Example: Ibuprofen 5-10 mg/kg/dose every 6-8 hours (maximum 40 mg/kg/day)

For 20 kg child receiving 200 mg every 6 hours:

- Individual dose: 200 mg ÷ 20 kg = 10 mg/kg (at upper limit)
- Daily dose: 200 mg × 4 doses = 800 mg
- Daily dose per kg: 800 mg ÷ 20 kg = 40 mg/kg (at maximum)

This dosing is at the maximum safe limits—no additional doses can be given without exceeding safety guidelines.

Age-Specific Dose Modifications

Some medications require dose adjustments based on age in addition to weight. Neonates and infants often need reduced doses due to immature organ function, while adolescents may need adult-level doses despite lower weights.

Always consult age-specific dosing guidelines when available, and verify that weight-based calculations are appropriate for the patient's developmental stage.

Case Study Applications

Case Study 1: Febrile Infant Management

Six-month-old Sarah Johnson weighs 8 kg and has a fever of 102.5°F. Her pediatrician prescribes acetaminophen 15 mg/kg every 4 hours as needed for fever.

Calculate individual dose: 8 kg × 15 mg/kg = 120 mg per dose

Available suspension: 80 mg per 2.5 mL (0.8 mL per dose unit)

Calculate volume needed: 120 mg × (2.5 mL / 80 mg) = 3.75 mL per dose

Verify maximum daily dosing: Maximum: 8 kg × 75 mg/kg/day = 600 mg/day If given every 4 hours (6 doses): 120 mg × 6 = 720 mg

This exceeds maximum daily dose—recommend spacing doses every 6 hours maximum: 120 mg × 4 doses = 480 mg/day (within safe limits)

Provide clear instructions: "Give 3.75 mL (3¾ mL) by mouth every 6 hours as needed for fever. Do not exceed 4 doses in 24 hours."

Case Study 2: Pediatric Pneumonia Treatment

Three-year-old Marcus Williams weighs 15 kg and needs amoxicillin for pneumonia. The prescribed dose is 80 mg/kg/day divided every 8 hours.

Calculate total daily dose: 15 kg × 80 mg/kg/day = 1,200 mg/day

Calculate individual dose: 1,200 mg/day ÷ 3 doses/day = 400 mg per dose

Available suspension: 250 mg per 5 mL

Calculate volume per dose: 400 mg × (5 mL / 250 mg) = 8 mL per dose

Verify dose safety: Reference range: 25-90 mg/kg/day for pneumonia Prescribed dose: 80 mg/kg/day (within safe range)

Duration: Complete 10-day course as prescribed

Instructions: "Give 8 mL by mouth every 8 hours for 10 days. Complete all medication even if symptoms improve."

Case Study 3: Emergency Department Pain Management

Eight-year-old Emma Rodriguez weighs 25 kg and needs morphine for pain from a femur fracture. The physician orders morphine 0.1 mg/kg IV every 4 hours as needed.

Calculate dose: 25 kg × 0.1 mg/kg = 2.5 mg per dose

Available concentration: 10 mg/mL

Calculate volume: 2.5 mg × (1 mL / 10 mg) = 0.25 mL per dose

Verify dose safety: Pediatric morphine range: 0.05-0.2 mg/kg/dose Prescribed dose: 0.1 mg/kg (within safe range)

Maximum frequency: Every 4 hours Maximum daily doses: 6 doses (if given consistently)

Administer slowly IV push over 2-3 minutes and monitor for respiratory depression, especially with first dose.

Body Surface Area Calculations

BSA Formula Applications

Body surface area calculations provide more accurate dosing for certain high-risk medications, particularly chemotherapy agents and some cardiac medications.

Example: Child height 100 cm, weight 20 kg

$BSA = \sqrt{[(100 \times 20) \div 3{,}600]} = \sqrt{[2{,}000 \div 3{,}600]} = \sqrt{0.556} = 0.75 \text{ m}^2$

For medication dosed at 30 mg/m²: 0.75 m² × 30 mg/m² = 22.5 mg

Nomogram Usage

BSA nomograms provide visual lookup tools that eliminate calculation complexity while maintaining accuracy. Place a straight edge connecting height and weight columns to find BSA intersection.

Always double-check nomogram readings, especially when measurements fall between marked lines. Small reading errors can lead to significant dosing mistakes.

BSA vs. Weight-Based Dosing

Use BSA calculations when specifically prescribed or when protocols require them. Most routine pediatric medications use weight-based dosing, which is simpler and equally effective for standard therapeutics.

BSA calculations typically apply to:

- Chemotherapy protocols
- Some cardiac medications
- Certain investigational drugs
- Specialized pediatric intensive care medications

Age-Specific Volume Limitations

Oral Medication Volume Considerations

Pediatric patients have limited ability to swallow large volumes of liquid medications. Consider practical administration limitations when calculating liquid doses.

Age-based volume guidelines:

- Infants (0-12 months): 5 mL maximum per dose
- Toddlers (1-3 years): 10 mL maximum per dose
- School age (4-11 years): 15-20 mL maximum per dose
- Adolescents (12+ years): Adult volumes acceptable

When calculated volumes exceed these limits, consider:

- Higher concentration formulations
- Dose division into multiple administrations
- Alternative routes (IV, IM)
- Tablet formulations for appropriate ages

Injectable Volume Restrictions

Pediatric injectable volume limitations are more stringent than oral limitations due to injection site capacity and patient comfort.

Intramuscular injection limits:

- Neonates/infants: 0.5 mL maximum
- Toddlers: 1 mL maximum
- School age: 1-2 mL maximum (depending on muscle mass)
- Adolescents: 2-3 mL maximum

Subcutaneous injection limits:

- All pediatric ages: 0.5-1 mL maximum per site

When volumes exceed these limits, use multiple injection sites or consider alternative routes.

Pediatric Emergency Calculations

Time-Critical Dosing

Pediatric emergencies require immediate, accurate calculations under extreme stress. Practice these calculations regularly to build automaticity when seconds matter.

Common emergency calculations:

- Epinephrine 0.01 mg/kg (0.1 mL/kg of 1:10,000) for cardiac arrest
- Adenosine 0.1 mg/kg (maximum 6 mg first dose) for SVT
- Atropine 0.02 mg/kg (minimum 0.1 mg) for bradycardia

Resuscitation Medication Preparation

Prepare emergency medications in standardized concentrations when possible to reduce calculation complexity during resuscitation efforts.

Example standardized preparation:

- Mix 6 mg adenosine in 60 mL normal saline = 0.1 mg/mL
- For any weight child: Give 1 mL/kg IV push for 0.1 mg/kg dose

This approach eliminates calculation needs during emergencies while maintaining accurate dosing.

Team Communication During Calculations

Emergency situations require clear communication of calculations to team members. Always state:

- Patient weight
- Dose calculation (mg/kg × weight = total dose)
- Volume calculation
- Verification of calculation

Example: "Patient weighs 20 kg. Epinephrine dose is 0.01 mg/kg times 20 kg equals 0.2 mg. Using 1:10,000 concentration, give 2 mL IV push."

Clinical Excellence: Pediatric Dosing Mastery

Pediatric medication calculations demand the highest level of mathematical precision and clinical judgment in nursing practice. Children's unique physiologic characteristics, narrow therapeutic windows, and limited ability to communicate adverse effects make calculation accuracy a matter of life and death in ways that exceed even critical care adult medication calculations.

Your mastery of weight-based dosing principles, safe dose range verification, and age-appropriate administration techniques enables you to provide safe, effective medication therapy across the entire pediatric population from premature neonates to adolescents approaching adult size.

The complexity of pediatric calculations—involving weight conversions, dose range verification, volume limitations, and emergency time pressures—requires systematic approaches and consistent practice to maintain competency. These skills distinguish pediatric nurses and other child-focused practitioners as specialists capable of managing the unique challenges of caring for developing patients.

Each calculation you perform for a pediatric patient represents a sacred trust from families who depend on your expertise to protect their most precious relationships. This responsibility makes pediatric calculation mastery both professionally essential and deeply meaningful.

Key Learning Points

- Pediatric physiology creates unique medication vulnerabilities requiring weight-based dosing with exceptional calculation accuracy
- Weight conversion accuracy forms the foundation for all subsequent pediatric medication calculations
- Safe dose range verification prevents both underdosing and overdosing in populations with narrow therapeutic windows
- Age-specific volume limitations require consideration of practical administration constraints alongside mathematical accuracy
- Emergency pediatric calculations demand automaticity and systematic approaches for time-critical medication administration

Chapter 8: Critical Care and High-Alert Medications

Critical care environments demand split-second decisions with life-or-death consequences. Here, medication calculations transcend routine mathematical exercises to become tools for hemodynamic rescue, cardiac stabilization, and physiologic support in patients whose organ systems teeter on the edge of failure. The medications you calculate in these settings—vasoactive drips, cardiac drugs, sedation protocols—can restore normal physiology or, if calculated incorrectly, precipitate catastrophic complications that end lives within minutes.

High-alert medications carry designation from The Joint Commission and Institute for Safe Medication Practices precisely because calculation errors result in severe patient harm or death. These medications demand heightened vigilance, mandatory double-checking, and calculation accuracy that leaves no room for mathematical approximation or clinical guesswork.

Understanding Critical Care Pharmacology

Vasoactive Medication Principles

Vasoactive medications directly affect blood vessel diameter and cardiac function, influencing blood pressure, heart rate, and tissue perfusion. These drugs work within minutes of administration and require continuous monitoring because therapeutic effects and toxic effects often differ by small concentration changes.

Vasopressors constrict blood vessels and increase cardiac contractility, raising blood pressure in patients with shock or hypotension. Common vasopressors include norepinephrine, epinephrine, dopamine, and phenylephrine.

Vasodilators relax blood vessel walls, reducing blood pressure and cardiac workload in patients with hypertensive emergencies or heart failure. Examples include nicardipine, clevidipine, and nitroglycerin.

Inotropes primarily affect cardiac contractility, strengthening heart muscle contractions to improve cardiac output. Dobutamine and milrinone represent commonly used inotropic agents.

Concentration-Dependent Effects

Many critical care medications produce different physiologic effects at different dose ranges. Dopamine exemplifies this complexity:

- Low doses (2-5 mcg/kg/min): Renal and mesenteric vasodilation
- Moderate doses (5-10 mcg/kg/min): Cardiac stimulation and increased contractility
- High doses (10-20 mcg/kg/min): Vasoconstriction and increased blood pressure

These dose-dependent effects require precise calculations to achieve desired therapeutic goals while avoiding unwanted effects.

Time-Sensitive Titration Requirements

Critical care medications often require frequent dose adjustments based on patient response. Titration protocols specify how quickly doses can be increased or decreased and what parameters guide these changes.

Example titration protocol: "Increase norepinephrine by 2-4 mcg/minute every 5 minutes until systolic blood pressure >90 mmHg or maximum dose 30 mcg/minute"

This protocol requires you to calculate new infusion rates quickly and accurately while monitoring patient response continuously.

Dopamine and Norepinephrine Calculations

Standard Concentration Preparations

Critical care units typically use standardized concentrations for vasoactive medications to reduce calculation complexity and error risk. Common standardizations include:

Dopamine: 400 mg in 250 mL (1,600 mcg/mL) or 800 mg in 250 mL (3,200 mcg/mL) Norepinephrine: 4 mg in 250 mL (16 mcg/mL) or 8 mg in 250 mL (32 mcg/mL)

These standardizations allow development of simplified calculation methods and dosing charts that reduce error risk during emergency situations.

Weight-Based Dosing Calculations

Most vasoactive medications dose according to patient weight, typically expressed as mcg/kg/minute. These calculations require conversion from mcg/kg/minute to mL/hour for infusion pump programming.

Basic calculation setup: (Dose in mcg/kg/min × Weight in kg × 60 min/hr) ÷ Concentration in mcg/mL = mL/hr

Example: Dopamine 10 mcg/kg/min for 70 kg patient using 1,600 mcg/mL concentration

Step 1: Calculate total mcg/minute: 10 mcg/kg/min × 70 kg = 700 mcg/min Step 2: Convert to mcg/hour: 700 mcg/min × 60 min/hr = 42,000 mcg/hr Step 3: Convert to mL/hr: 42,000 mcg/hr ÷ 1,600 mcg/mL = 26.25 mL/hr

Program infusion pump for 26.3 mL/hr (rounded to nearest tenth).

Dose Range Calculations

Physicians often order vasoactive medications within dose ranges, allowing nurses to titrate based on patient response. Calculate both minimum and maximum infusion rates to establish titration boundaries.

Example: Norepinephrine 0.05-0.3 mcg/kg/min for 80 kg patient using 16 mcg/mL concentration

Minimum dose calculation: 0.05 mcg/kg/min × 80 kg × 60 min/hr ÷ 16 mcg/mL = 15 mL/hr

Maximum dose calculation: 0.3 mcg/kg/min × 80 kg × 60 min/hr ÷ 16 mcg/mL = 90 mL/hr

Titration range: 15-90 mL/hr on infusion pump

Titration Increment Calculations

Titration protocols specify dose increases in mcg/kg/min or total mcg/min. Convert these increments to mL/hr changes for practical implementation.

Example: "Increase norepinephrine by 0.05 mcg/kg/min every 5 minutes as needed"

For 80 kg patient with 16 mcg/mL concentration: 0.05 mcg/kg/min × 80 kg × 60 min/hr ÷ 16 mcg/mL = 15 mL/hr

Increase pump rate by 15 mL/hr with each titration step.

Heparin Protocol Management

Weight-Based Heparin Protocols

Therapeutic heparin administration follows weight-based protocols designed to achieve target partial thromboplastin times (PTT) while minimizing bleeding risk. These protocols specify initial dosing, adjustment criteria, and maximum dose limits.

Typical protocol components:

- Initial bolus: 80 units/kg IV push
- Initial infusion: 18 units/kg/hour
- Adjustment increments based on PTT results
- Maximum infusion rate limits

Protocol Calculation Applications

Example protocol for 75 kg patient:

Initial bolus calculation: 75 kg × 80 units/kg = 6,000 units IV push

Using 5,000 units/mL concentration: 6,000 units ÷ 5,000 units/mL = 1.2 mL IV push

Initial infusion calculation: 75 kg × 18 units/kg/hr = 1,350 units/hr

Using standard concentration 25,000 units in 250 mL (100 units/mL): 1,350 units/hr ÷ 100 units/mL = 13.5 mL/hr

PTT-Based Dose Adjustments

Heparin protocols include adjustment tables based on PTT results. These adjustments require recalculation of infusion rates to maintain therapeutic anticoagulation.

Example adjustment: "If PTT 46-70 seconds, increase rate by 2 units/kg/hr"

For 75 kg patient: 2 units/kg/hr × 75 kg = 150 units/hr increase

New infusion rate: 1,350 + 150 = 1,500 units/hr New pump setting: 1,500 units/hr ÷ 100 units/mL = 15 mL/hr

Monitoring and Safety Parameters

Heparin protocols require frequent PTT monitoring and dose adjustments. Calculate new rates promptly when lab results become available to maintain therapeutic levels.

Safety considerations:

- Maximum dose limits prevent excessive anticoagulation
- Hold parameters specify when to stop infusions
- Reversal protocols guide emergency management of bleeding complications

Insulin Drip Calculations

Critical Care Insulin Protocols

Intensive care patients often require IV insulin infusions to maintain tight glycemic control. These protocols specify target glucose ranges, initial dosing, and adjustment criteria based on blood glucose trends.

Common protocol structure:

- Initial rate based on blood glucose level
- Hourly rate adjustments based on glucose changes
- Target range: 140-180 mg/dL (varies by institution)
- Maximum rate limits for safety

Protocol Implementation Calculations

Example protocol for patient with blood glucose 250 mg/dL:

Initial rate determination from protocol table: Blood glucose 201-250 mg/dL: Start insulin at 2 units/hr

Using standard concentration 100 units in 100 mL normal saline (1 unit/mL): 2 units/hr ÷ 1 unit/mL = 2 mL/hr

Adjustment Calculations

Insulin protocols require frequent rate adjustments based on glucose trends and current rates. These calculations must be performed quickly to maintain target glucose ranges.

Example adjustment scenario: Current rate: 4 units/hr Current glucose: 200 mg/dL
Previous glucose: 180 mg/dL (increase of 20 mg/dL)

Protocol instruction: "If glucose increased by 20-40 mg/dL, increase rate by 1 unit/hr"

New rate: 4 + 1 = 5 units/hr New pump setting: 5 mL/hr

Hypoglycemia Management

Insulin protocols include specific instructions for managing hypoglycemia, including when to stop insulin, when to give dextrose, and when to restart insulin infusions.

Example hypoglycemia protocol:

- Glucose <70 mg/dL: Stop insulin, give dextrose 25 g (50 mL D50W) IV
- Recheck glucose in 15 minutes
- Restart insulin at half previous rate when glucose >100 mg/dL

Sedation and Analgesia Calculations

Continuous Sedation Protocols

Critical care patients often require continuous sedation to maintain comfort and synchrony with mechanical ventilation. Sedation calculations involve weight-based dosing with frequent adjustments based on sedation scores.

Common sedation medications:

- Propofol: 5-50 mcg/kg/min
- Midazolam: 0.02-0.1 mg/kg/hr
- Dexmedetomidine: 0.2-0.7 mcg/kg/hr

Propofol Calculation Examples

Propofol requires careful calculation due to high lipid content and potential for rapid onset/offset effects.

Example: 70 kg patient requiring propofol 20 mcg/kg/min

Using standard concentration 10 mg/mL (10,000 mcg/mL):

Calculate total mcg/min: 70 kg × 20 mcg/kg/min = 1,400 mcg/min
Convert to mcg/hr: 1,400 mcg/min × 60 min/hr = 84,000 mcg/hr
Convert to mL/hr: 84,000 mcg/hr ÷ 10,000 mcg/mL = 8.4 mL/hr

Analgesia Protocol Calculations

Pain management in critical care often involves continuous opioid infusions with bolus dosing capabilities for breakthrough pain.

Example fentanyl protocol:

- Continuous rate: 0.5-2 mcg/kg/hr
- Bolus dose: 0.5-1 mcg/kg every 15 minutes as needed
- Maximum hourly dose including boluses: 4 mcg/kg/hr

For 80 kg patient: Continuous rate: 80 kg × 1 mcg/kg/hr = 80 mcg/hr
Bolus dose: 80 kg × 0.5 mcg/kg = 40 mcg per bolus Maximum hourly: 80 kg × 4 mcg/kg/hr = 320 mcg/hr

Using 50 mcg/mL concentration: Continuous: 80 mcg/hr ÷ 50 mcg/mL = 1.6 mL/hr Bolus: 40 mcg ÷ 50 mcg/mL = 0.8 mL per bolus

Case Study Applications

Case Study 1: Septic Shock Management

Maria Santos, a 55-year-old woman with pneumonia, develops septic shock requiring vasopressor support. She weighs 60 kg with blood pressure 75/40 mmHg despite fluid resuscitation.

Physician orders: Norepinephrine 0.1 mcg/kg/min, titrate by 0.05 mcg/kg/min every 5 minutes to maintain systolic BP >90 mmHg, maximum dose 0.5 mcg/kg/min.

Using 8 mg in 250 mL concentration (32 mcg/mL):

Initial dose calculation: 0.1 mcg/kg/min × 60 kg × 60 min/hr ÷ 32 mcg/mL = 11.25 mL/hr

Titration increment: 0.05 mcg/kg/min × 60 kg × 60 min/hr ÷ 32 mcg/mL = 5.6 mL/hr (round to 6 mL/hr)

Maximum dose: 0.5 mcg/kg/min × 60 kg × 60 min/hr ÷ 32 mcg/mL = 56.25 mL/hr

Titration plan: Start at 11 mL/hr, increase by 6 mL/hr every 5 minutes as needed, maximum 56 mL/hr.

Case Study 2: Post-Cardiac Surgery Patient

Robert Kim, a 68-year-old man, returns from cardiac surgery requiring multiple vasoactive drips for hemodynamic support. He weighs 75 kg.

Current orders:

- Epinephrine 0.05 mcg/kg/min
- Milrinone 0.375 mcg/kg/min
- Norepinephrine 0.15 mcg/kg/min

Calculate all three infusion rates:

Epinephrine (1 mg in 250 mL = 4 mcg/mL): 0.05 mcg/kg/min × 75 kg × 60 min/hr ÷ 4 mcg/mL = 56.25 mL/hr

Milrinone (20 mg in 100 mL = 200 mcg/mL): 0.375 mcg/kg/min × 75 kg × 60 min/hr ÷ 200 mcg/mL = 8.4 mL/hr

Norepinephrine (8 mg in 250 mL = 32 mcg/mL): 0.15 mcg/kg/min × 75 kg × 60 min/hr ÷ 32 mcg/mL = 21.1 mL/hr

Monitor hemodynamic parameters continuously and titrate per protocol based on cardiac output, blood pressure, and urine output.

Case Study 3: Diabetic Ketoacidosis Management

Jennifer Lopez, a 25-year-old woman with type 1 diabetes, presents in DKA with blood glucose 450 mg/dL. She weighs 55 kg.

Insulin protocol orders:

- Initial rate: 0.1 units/kg/hr
- Adjust every hour based on glucose decline and target rate of 50-75 mg/dL/hr decrease
- Target glucose 200-250 mg/dL before transitioning to subcutaneous insulin

Initial insulin calculation: 0.1 units/kg/hr × 55 kg = 5.5 units/hr

Using 100 units in 100 mL concentration: 5.5 units/hr ÷ 1 unit/mL = 5.5 mL/hr

Hourly monitoring plan:

- Check glucose every hour
- Calculate glucose change from previous hour
- Adjust rate per protocol to maintain 50-75 mg/dL/hr decline
- Monitor electrolytes and adjust IV fluids accordingly

Double-Check Procedures and Safety

Independent Verification Requirements

High-alert medications require independent verification by two qualified nurses before administration. This process includes:

1. Independent calculation by both nurses
2. Comparison of calculation results
3. Verification of medication concentration
4. Confirmation of pump programming
5. Documentation of double-check completion

Both nurses must initial documentation confirming independent verification was completed.

Calculation Method Verification

Use different calculation methods for verification when possible. If the primary nurse uses dimensional analysis, the verifying nurse might use ratio-proportion or formula method to confirm accuracy.

Example verification: Primary calculation: 0.1 mcg/kg/min × 70 kg × 60 ÷ 16 mcg/mL = 26.25 mL/hr

Verification using ratio-proportion: 0.1 mcg/kg/min × 70 kg = 7 mcg/min = 420 mcg/hr 16 mcg : 1 mL = 420 mcg : X mL X = 420 ÷ 16 = 26.25 mL/hr ✓

Technology Integration and Smart Pumps

Smart pumps with drug libraries provide additional safety layers for high-alert medications. These systems:

- Verify dose ranges are within established limits
- Calculate infusion rates automatically when programmed with doses
- Provide alerts for potentially dangerous rates or doses
- Document administration automatically

Always verify that smart pump calculations match your manual calculations before starting infusions.

Life-Saving Precision: Critical Care Excellence

Critical care medication calculations represent the pinnacle of nursing mathematical responsibility. In these environments, your calculation accuracy directly determines whether patients survive catastrophic illness or succumb to organ failure. The medications you calculate and administer—vasopressors, insulin drips, sedation protocols—maintain life itself when normal physiology fails.

The complexity of critical care calculations demands mastery that extends beyond mathematical computation to include deep understanding of pharmacology, patient physiology, and protocol interpretation. Your ability to calculate quickly and accurately under extreme pressure, while maintaining awareness of drug interactions and patient response patterns, distinguishes expert critical care practitioners from those who struggle with basic ICU responsibilities.

Each calculation you perform in critical care settings carries weight that exceeds routine medication administration. These are not simply numerical exercises—they are clinical interventions that support cardiac function, maintain blood pressure, control blood glucose, and provide comfort to patients fighting for survival.

Your expertise with these calculations enables you to function as a trusted member of critical care teams where physicians rely on your mathematical competency and clinical judgment to implement complex therapeutic regimens that save lives every day.

Key Learning Points

- Vasoactive medication calculations require understanding of dose-dependent effects and precise weight-based dosing techniques
- Heparin protocol management integrates initial dosing calculations with ongoing adjustments based on laboratory monitoring
- Insulin drip calculations demand frequent rate adjustments to maintain target glucose ranges while preventing hypoglycemia
- Sedation calculations balance patient comfort with safety considerations through systematic titration approaches

- High-alert medication safety requires independent verification procedures and technology integration for error prevention

Chapter 9: Complex Multi-Step Clinical Scenarios

Real-world nursing practice rarely involves isolated medication calculations. Instead, you face complex clinical situations requiring multiple interrelated calculations, clinical judgment integration, and adaptation to changing patient conditions. These scenarios test your ability to synthesize mathematical skills with nursing knowledge while managing time pressures and competing priorities that characterize modern healthcare environments.

Complex scenarios force you beyond algorithmic calculation approaches toward clinical reasoning that considers patient-specific factors, equipment limitations, medication interactions, and safety protocols simultaneously. This chapter develops the advanced problem-solving skills needed to excel in challenging clinical situations across diverse healthcare settings.

Medical-Surgical Unit Case Studies

Case Study 1: Post-Operative Infection Management

Dorothy Williams, a 72-year-old woman, underwent hip replacement surgery three days ago and now shows signs of surgical site infection. She weighs 58 kg, has normal kidney function, and has no known drug allergies. The physician orders multiple interventions requiring coordinated calculations.

Current Orders:

- Vancomycin 15 mg/kg IV every 12 hours
- Normal saline 1,000 mL with potassium chloride 20 mEq IV over 8 hours
- Acetaminophen 650 mg PO every 6 hours for pain
- Docusate sodium 100 mg PO twice daily for constipation prevention

88

Calculation Sequence:

Vancomycin Dosing: Step 1: Calculate dose: 58 kg × 15 mg/kg = 870 mg every 12 hours Step 2: Available concentration: 500 mg/100 mL, infuse over 60 minutes Step 3: Volume calculation: 870 mg × (100 mL/500 mg) = 174 mL Step 4: Infusion rate: 174 mL ÷ 1 hour = 174 mL/hr

IV Fluid with Additive: Step 1: Verify potassium concentration: 20 mEq in 1,000 mL = 20 mEq/L Step 2: Check maximum concentration guidelines: 40 mEq/L maximum (safe) Step 3: Calculate infusion rate: 1,000 mL ÷ 8 hours = 125 mL/hr

Oral Medications: Acetaminophen: Available as 325 mg tablets 650 mg ÷ 325 mg/tablet = 2 tablets every 6 hours

Docusate: Available as 100 mg capsules (no calculation needed)

Clinical Considerations:

- Schedule vancomycin to avoid overlap with other nephrotoxic medications
- Monitor IV site carefully with potassium-containing fluids
- Track total daily acetaminophen to avoid exceeding 3,000 mg/day limit
- Coordinate timing to minimize pill burden for patient

Case Study 2: Diabetes Management with Complications

Frank Rodriguez, a 65-year-old man with type 2 diabetes, presents with hyperglycemic hyperosmolar syndrome. He weighs 85 kg and requires complex fluid and insulin management.

Current Orders:

- Normal saline 500 mL bolus over 1 hour, then 250 mL/hr × 4 hours
- Regular insulin 0.1 units/kg/hr continuous IV infusion

- Potassium chloride 40 mEq in 1,000 mL normal saline over 6 hours (when serum K+ <5.0)
- Sliding scale insulin coverage in addition to continuous infusion

Calculation Sequence:

Fluid Resuscitation: Initial bolus: 500 mL over 1 hour = 500 mL/hr Maintenance: 250 mL/hr × 4 hours = 1,000 mL Total first 5 hours: 500 + 1,000 = 1,500 mL

Continuous Insulin: 85 kg × 0.1 units/kg/hr = 8.5 units/hr Using 100 units in 100 mL: 8.5 units/hr = 8.5 mL/hr

Potassium Replacement: 40 mEq in 1,000 mL = 40 mEq/L concentration Infusion rate: 1,000 mL ÷ 6 hours = 167 mL/hr Potassium delivery rate: 40 mEq ÷ 6 hours = 6.7 mEq/hr

Sliding Scale Addition: Current glucose: 350 mg/dL Sliding scale: 4 units subcutaneous for glucose 301-350 mg/dL Administer 4 units subcutaneous plus continue 8.5 units/hr IV

Clinical Monitoring:

- Check glucose hourly and adjust continuous insulin per protocol
- Monitor electrolytes every 4 hours
- Track fluid balance carefully to avoid overload
- Coordinate timing of subcutaneous and IV insulin

ICU/Critical Care Cases

Case Study 3: Multi-Organ Failure Support

Patricia Chen, a 45-year-old woman with sepsis, develops multi-organ failure requiring multiple vasoactive drips, renal replacement therapy, and sedation. She weighs 70 kg.

Current Orders:

- Norepinephrine 0.2 mcg/kg/min, titrate to MAP >65 mmHg
- Vasopressin 2.4 units/hr (fixed dose)
- Propofol 30 mcg/kg/min for sedation
- Fentanyl 1 mcg/kg/hr for analgesia
- Continuous renal replacement therapy at 2,000 mL/hr

Calculation Sequence:

Norepinephrine (8 mg in 250 mL = 32 mcg/mL): 0.2 mcg/kg/min ×
70 kg × 60 min/hr ÷ 32 mcg/mL = 26.25 mL/hr

Vasopressin (20 units in 100 mL = 0.2 units/mL): 2.4 units/hr ÷ 0.2
units/mL = 12 mL/hr

Propofol (10 mg/mL = 10,000 mcg/mL): 30 mcg/kg/min × 70 kg ×
60 min/hr ÷ 10,000 mcg/mL = 12.6 mL/hr

Fentanyl (50 mcg/mL): 1 mcg/kg/hr × 70 kg ÷ 50 mcg/mL = 1.4
mL/hr

Fluid Balance Considerations: Drug delivery fluids: 26.25 + 12 +
12.6 + 1.4 = 52.25 mL/hr CRRT removal rate: 2,000 mL/hr Net fluid
removal: 2,000 - 52.25 = 1,947.75 mL/hr

Clinical Integration:

- Monitor MAP continuously and titrate norepinephrine
  accordingly
- Assess sedation level every 2 hours and adjust propofol
- Coordinate with nephrology for CRRT management
- Track cumulative fluid balance including all sources

Case Study 4: Post-Cardiac Surgery Recovery

Michael Thompson, a 62-year-old man, returns from coronary artery bypass surgery requiring hemodynamic support and anticoagulation management. He weighs 80 kg.

Current Orders:

- Epinephrine 0.03 mcg/kg/min
- Milrinone loading dose 50 mcg/kg over 10 minutes, then 0.5 mcg/kg/min
- Heparin per protocol: 80 units/kg bolus, then 18 units/kg/hr
- Nitroglycerin 10-20 mcg/min for afterload reduction

Calculation Sequence:

Epinephrine (1 mg in 250 mL = 4 mcg/mL): 0.03 mcg/kg/min × 80 kg × 60 min/hr ÷ 4 mcg/mL = 36 mL/hr

Milrinone Loading: 50 mcg/kg × 80 kg = 4,000 mcg = 4 mg Using 1 mg/mL concentration: 4 mg ÷ 1 mg/mL = 4 mL over 10 minutes Loading rate: 4 mL ÷ (10/60) hours = 24 mL/hr for 10 minutes

Milrinone Maintenance (200 mcg/mL): 0.5 mcg/kg/min × 80 kg × 60 min/hr ÷ 200 mcg/mL = 12 mL/hr

Heparin Protocol: Bolus: 80 units/kg × 80 kg = 6,400 units IV push Infusion: 18 units/kg/hr × 80 kg = 1,440 units/hr Using 25,000 units in 250 mL: 1,440 units/hr ÷ 100 units/mL = 14.4 mL/hr

Nitroglycerin (50 mg in 250 mL = 200 mcg/mL): Starting dose: 10 mcg/min × 60 min/hr ÷ 200 mcg/mL = 3 mL/hr

Titration Planning:

- Monitor cardiac output and adjust milrinone accordingly
- Titrate nitroglycerin based on blood pressure and SVR
- Follow heparin protocol for PTT-based adjustments
- Assess for weaning epinephrine as cardiac function improves

Pediatric/NICU Cases

Case Study 5: Premature Infant Respiratory Support

Baby Johnson, born at 28 weeks gestation, weighs 1.2 kg and requires mechanical ventilation with medication support for respiratory distress syndrome.

Current Orders:

- Caffeine citrate loading dose 20 mg/kg IV over 30 minutes
- Caffeine citrate maintenance 5 mg/kg/day IV daily
- Dexamethasone 0.15 mg/kg/dose IV every 12 hours × 3 days
- D10W with calcium gluconate 200 mg/kg/day continuous IV

Calculation Sequence:

Caffeine Loading: 20 mg/kg × 1.2 kg = 24 mg loading dose Using 20 mg/mL concentration: 24 mg ÷ 20 mg/mL = 1.2 mL Infusion rate: 1.2 mL ÷ 0.5 hours = 2.4 mL/hr for 30 minutes

Caffeine Maintenance: 5 mg/kg/day × 1.2 kg = 6 mg daily Volume: 6 mg ÷ 20 mg/mL = 0.3 mL daily

Dexamethasone: 0.15 mg/kg × 1.2 kg = 0.18 mg every 12 hours Using 4 mg/mL concentration: 0.18 mg ÷ 4 mg/mL = 0.045 mL

Calcium Gluconate Continuous: 200 mg/kg/day × 1.2 kg = 240 mg/day 240 mg/day ÷ 24 hours = 10 mg/hr Using 100 mg/mL: 10 mg/hr ÷ 100 mg/mL = 0.1 mL/hr

Fluid Management: Total IV fluids needed: 120 mL/kg/day × 1.2 kg = 144 mL/day = 6 mL/hr Medication fluids: 0.1 mL/hr calcium + daily caffeine volume Maintenance D10W: Adjust to meet total fluid needs

Clinical Considerations:

- Monitor respiratory status closely during steroid course
- Watch for caffeine toxicity signs (tachycardia, irritability)
- Track fluid balance precisely in this small patient
- Coordinate timing to minimize handling

Emergency Department Cases

Case Study 6: Multi-Trauma Resuscitation

James Wilson, a 25-year-old man, arrives following motorcycle accident with multiple injuries. He weighs 75 kg and requires immediate resuscitation.

Current Orders:

- Lactated Ringer's 2 L bolus as fast as possible
- Type and crossmatch for 6 units packed red blood cells
- Morphine 0.1 mg/kg IV every 4 hours for pain
- Cefazolin 2 g IV every 8 hours for open fracture prophylaxis
- Tetanus toxoid 0.5 mL IM × 1 dose

Calculation Sequence:

Fluid Resuscitation: 2,000 mL as fast as IV access allows Using 14-gauge IVs with pressure bags for maximum flow

Morphine Pain Management: 0.1 mg/kg × 75 kg = 7.5 mg every 4 hours Using 10 mg/mL: 7.5 mg ÷ 10 mg/mL = 0.75 mL IV push

Cefazolin Prophylaxis: 2 g every 8 hours (standard adult dose, no calculation needed) Mix in 50 mL normal saline, infuse over 30 minutes Infusion rate: 50 mL ÷ 0.5 hours = 100 mL/hr

Clinical Priorities:

- Establish large-bore IV access immediately
- Monitor vital signs continuously during resuscitation
- Prepare for potential blood transfusion needs

- Coordinate with surgical team for definitive management

Equipment Limitations and Adaptations

Syringe Pump Limitations

Some critical care medications require syringe pumps due to concentration or compatibility issues. These pumps typically accommodate 20-60 mL syringes, affecting preparation calculations.

Example: Norepinephrine for 70 kg patient at 0.1 mcg/kg/min using 60 mL syringe pump

Standard concentration (8 mg in 250 mL) would require frequent syringe changes.

Alternative preparation for syringe pump: Mix 8 mg norepinephrine in 60 mL = 133.3 mcg/mL

Calculate infusion rate: 0.1 mcg/kg/min × 70 kg × 60 min/hr ÷ 133.3 mcg/mL = 3.15 mL/hr

Syringe duration: 60 mL ÷ 3.15 mL/hr = 19 hours

IV Access Limitations

Peripheral IV gauge limitations affect infusion rate capabilities and medication compatibility decisions.

22-gauge IV maximum flow rates:

- Crystalloid solutions: ~75 mL/min gravity, ~150 mL/hr pump maximum
- Blood products: Slower rates due to viscosity
- Vesicant medications: May require central access

Calculate whether planned infusions exceed IV capabilities and plan accordingly.

Pump Capability Constraints

Some medications require infusion rates that exceed standard pump capabilities or precision.

Example: Very low-dose vasopressin 0.5 units/hr Standard concentration (20 units in 100 mL = 0.2 units/mL): 0.5 units/hr ÷

0.2 units/mL = 2.5 mL/hr

Most pumps can deliver this rate accurately, but concentrations requiring rates <1 mL/hr may need dilution or specialized pumps.

Medication Reconciliation Scenarios

Transfer Between Units

Patients transferring between units often require medication reconciliation involving calculation verification and route conversions.

Example: ICU patient on propofol 20 mL/hr (10 mg/mL) concentration) transferring to step-down unit without continuous sedation capability.

Current dose: 20 mL/hr × 10 mg/mL = 200 mg/hr

Conversion to intermittent sedation:

- Lorazepam 2 mg IV every 4 hours (equivalent anxiolysis)
- Monitor sedation level and adjust frequency

Calculate propofol wean schedule:

- Decrease by 25% every 30 minutes
- Hour 1: 200 mg/hr → 150 mg/hr (15 mL/hr)
- Hour 1.5: 150 mg/hr → 112.5 mg/hr (11.3 mL/hr)
- Hour 2: 112.5 mg/hr → 84.4 mg/hr (8.4 mL/hr)

- Continue until discontinuation

Home Medication Conversion

Discharge planning requires converting hospital medications to home equivalents with dosing calculations.

Example: Patient receiving IV morphine 2 mg every 4 hours converting to oral pain management.

Morphine IV to PO conversion ratio: 1:3 (oral dose is 3× IV dose) Current IV dose: 2 mg every 4 hours = 12 mg/day IV Equivalent oral dose: 12 mg × 3 = 36 mg/day oral

Available oral morphine: 15 mg tablets Dosing schedule: 15 mg every 12 hours (30 mg/day - close approximation)

Provide patient education: "Take one 15 mg tablet by mouth every 12 hours for pain. Take with food to prevent stomach upset."

Time Management and Prioritization

Critical Timing Calculations

Emergency situations require rapid calculation prioritization based on medication urgency and patient acuity.

Priority levels for calculation urgency:

1. **Immediate (within 1 minute)**: Vasopressors, cardiac arrest drugs, emergency antidotes
2. **Urgent (within 5 minutes)**: Pain medications, sedation adjustments, insulin corrections
3. **Important (within 15 minutes)**: Antibiotics, routine medications, fluid adjustments
4. **Routine (within 30 minutes)**: Discharge medications, home care instructions

Workflow Organization Strategies

Systematic approaches reduce calculation errors under time pressure:

1. **Gather all information first**: Weight, allergies, current medications, laboratory values
2. **Identify critical calculations**: Start with life-threatening medication needs
3. **Use standardized methods**: Stick to familiar calculation approaches under pressure
4. **Double-check critical drugs**: High-alert medications require verification
5. **Document systematically**: Clear documentation prevents repeat calculations

Delegation and Verification

Complex patients require team coordination for calculation verification and medication administration.

Delegation principles:

- Licensed nurses verify all high-alert medication calculations
- Unlicensed personnel cannot perform medication calculations
- Student nurses require supervision for all calculations
- Pharmacists provide consultation for complex protocols

Quality Improvement and Error Prevention

Calculation Error Analysis

Understanding common error patterns helps prevent future mistakes:

Decimal point errors: Most dangerous and common

- Always use leading zeros (0.5 mg, not .5 mg)
- Avoid trailing zeros (5 mg, not 5.0 mg)
- Double-check decimal placement in complex calculations

Unit confusion: Second most common error type

- Maintain consistent units throughout calculations
- Convert to common units early in calculation process
- Verify final answer units make clinical sense

Setup errors: Proportion and formula mistakes

- Write out complete setups before calculating
- Use dimensional analysis for complex problems
- Verify relationships make logical sense

Systematic Verification Methods

Develop personal verification routines for consistent accuracy:

1. **Estimate first**: Does the calculated answer seem reasonable?
2. **Use different method**: Verify complex calculations with alternative approach
3. **Work backwards**: Multiply final answer back to original dose
4. **Check references**: Verify doses against reliable sources
5. **Seek consultation**: Ask colleagues or pharmacists when uncertain

Technology Integration for Safety

Modern healthcare technology provides calculation support while requiring verification skills:

Smart pump integration:

- Program patient weight accurately
- Select correct medication from drug library
- Verify pump calculations match manual calculations
- Monitor for pump alerts and warnings

Clinical decision support:

- Use institution-approved calculation apps
- Verify app results with manual calculations
- Maintain manual calculation skills for technology failures
- Document calculation sources when required

Professional Excellence: Mastering Clinical Complexity

Complex multi-step clinical scenarios represent the reality of modern nursing practice where isolated medication calculations rarely exist. Instead, you face interconnected clinical challenges requiring mathematical precision, clinical judgment, and systematic problem-solving under time pressure and competing priorities.

Your ability to navigate these complex scenarios—integrating multiple medication calculations with patient assessment, equipment limitations, and safety protocols—distinguishes expert practitioners from those who struggle with real-world clinical demands. Each scenario you master builds confidence and competence that transfers to similar situations throughout your career.

The mathematical skills you've developed throughout this workbook converge in these complex scenarios, creating opportunities to demonstrate comprehensive competency while protecting patient safety through systematic approaches to challenging clinical problems.

These scenarios prepare you for advanced practice roles where complex calculation skills combine with clinical expertise to provide life-saving interventions in critical situations. Your mastery of these challenging calculations enables you to function as a trusted team member capable of managing the most complex patients in any healthcare environment.

Key Learning Points

- Complex scenarios require integration of multiple calculation types with clinical judgment and safety considerations

- Medical-surgical cases combine routine calculations with patient-specific factors and monitoring requirements
- Critical care scenarios demand rapid, accurate calculations for life-supporting medications under extreme pressure
- Pediatric cases require specialized approaches that account for developmental physiology and safety considerations
- Equipment limitations and medication reconciliation add complexity that requires adaptive problem-solving skills

Chapter 10: NCLEX Preparation and Competency Testing

The NCLEX examination represents the culmination of your nursing education and the gateway to professional practice. Medication calculation questions appear throughout the exam, integrated with clinical scenarios that test your ability to apply mathematical skills in realistic patient care situations. Success requires not only calculation accuracy but also clinical judgment, test-taking strategies, and confidence under examination pressure.

This chapter provides the focused preparation needed to excel on NCLEX medication math questions while building the competency testing skills required throughout your nursing career. Every calculation you perform during licensure and employment competency testing reflects your commitment to patient safety and professional excellence.

Understanding NCLEX Medication Math Integration

Question Format Evolution

NCLEX medication calculation questions have evolved from isolated mathematical problems to integrated clinical scenarios requiring both calculation skills and nursing judgment. Modern exam questions embed calculations within patient care situations, testing your ability to synthesize mathematical competency with clinical reasoning.

Traditional format example: "A patient needs 250 mg of medication. Available tablets contain 125 mg each. How many tablets should the nurse give?"

Modern integrated format example: "A nurse is caring for a patient with pneumonia who has difficulty swallowing pills. The physician orders amoxicillin 500 mg every 8 hours. Available suspension contains 250 mg per 5 mL. The nurse should administer how many mL per dose?"

The modern format requires you to recognize calculation needs within clinical contexts while considering patient-specific factors that affect medication administration.

Next Generation NCLEX Enhancements

The Next Generation NCLEX introduces enhanced question formats that more closely mirror real-world clinical decision-making:

Case study questions: Extended scenarios with multiple related questions, including calculations integrated with assessment, planning, and evaluation.

Drag-and-drop calculations: Interactive formats where you move numbers or units to complete calculations visually.

Hot spot questions: Click on syringes, medication cups, or other measurement devices to indicate correct volumes.

Enhanced multiple choice: Questions with multiple correct answers requiring comprehensive understanding of calculation principles.

These formats test calculation skills within broader clinical reasoning frameworks rather than as isolated mathematical exercises.

Test-Taking Strategies for Calculation Questions

Systematic Problem Approach

Develop consistent approaches to calculation questions that work reliably under examination pressure:

Step 1: Read completely

- Read the entire question before starting calculations

- Identify what the question asks you to find
- Note any patient-specific information that affects dosing

Step 2: Extract key information

- Patient weight (for weight-based dosing)
- Prescribed dose and frequency
- Available medication strength and form
- Any special administration considerations

Step 3: Set up calculation systematically

- Use dimensional analysis for complex problems
- Write out complete setups before calculating
- Include units with all numbers

Step 4: Calculate carefully

- Work step-by-step without rushing
- Round appropriately for the medication type
- Include units in your final answer

Step 5: Verify reasonableness

- Does the answer make clinical sense?
- Is the volume or number of tablets reasonable?
- Double-check decimal point placement

Common Calculation Question Types

Oral medication calculations: Test basic proportion skills and tablet/liquid conversions. Strategy: Focus on setup accuracy and appropriate rounding for the medication form.

Injectable calculations: Include reconstitution, concentration conversions, and volume determinations. Strategy: Pay careful attention to concentration units and volume limitations.

IV calculations: Test flow rate determinations, time calculations, and pump programming. Strategy: Verify time units (minutes vs. hours) and use appropriate formulas.

Pediatric calculations: Combine weight-based dosing with age-appropriate considerations. Strategy: Always start with accurate weight conversion and verify safe dose ranges.

Critical care calculations: Integrate complex drip rate calculations with patient monitoring. Strategy: Use systematic approaches and verify units throughout multi-step calculations.

Error Recognition Strategies

NCLEX questions sometimes test your ability to identify calculation errors or unsafe practices:

- Recognize when calculated doses exceed safe ranges
- Identify decimal point errors in medication orders
- Spot unit conversion mistakes
- Recognize inappropriate rounding practices

Practice identifying errors in example calculations to build pattern recognition for examination scenarios.

Building Confidence Through Practice

Progressive Skill Building

Build confidence through systematic practice that mirrors your skill development throughout this workbook:

Foundation level: Review basic mathematical operations, unit conversions, and simple medication calculations until automatic.

Application level: Practice integrated scenarios that combine calculations with clinical decision-making.

Synthesis level: Work through complex, multi-step problems that require multiple calculation types.

Mastery level: Complete timed practice exams that simulate testing conditions and pressure.

Anxiety Management Techniques

Calculation anxiety affects many nursing students, but systematic preparation and anxiety management techniques build confidence:

Preparation strategies:

- Practice calculations daily, even briefly
- Use realistic practice questions and timing
- Review common formulas until memorized
- Practice with calculator types allowed on exams

During-exam strategies:

- Take deep breaths before starting calculation questions
- Write out setups completely before calculating
- Trust your preparation and systematic approaches
- Move on if stuck and return to difficult questions

Confidence-building exercises:

- Start practice sessions with problems you know you can solve
- Gradually increase complexity as confidence builds
- Track improvement over time to see progress
- Celebrate accuracy achievements

Comprehensive Practice Examinations

Practice Exam 1: Foundation Assessment

Question 1: A patient needs acetaminophen 650 mg. Available tablets contain 325 mg each. How many tablets should the nurse administer?

Question 2: A pediatric patient weighing 20 kg needs amoxicillin 40 mg/kg/day divided into three doses. How many mg should the patient receive per dose?

Question 3: An IV infusion of 1,000 mL normal saline should infuse over 8 hours. Calculate the infusion rate in mL/hr.

Question 4: A patient needs morphine 4 mg IV. Available concentration is 10 mg/mL. How many mL should the nurse draw up?

Question 5: Heparin is ordered at 25,000 units in 250 mL to infuse at 15 units/kg/hr for a 70 kg patient. Calculate the infusion rate in mL/hr.

Solutions and Rationales:

Question 1: 650 mg ÷ 325 mg/tablet = 2 tablets *Rationale: Simple proportion calculation. Verify: 2 × 325 = 650 mg ✓*

Question 2: Step 1: 20 kg × 40 mg/kg/day = 800 mg/day Step 2: 800 mg/day ÷ 3 doses = 267 mg per dose *Rationale: Weight-based daily dose divided by frequency*

Question 3: 1,000 mL ÷ 8 hours = 125 mL/hr *Rationale: Basic infusion rate calculation. Common formula: Volume ÷ Time*

Question 4: 4 mg ÷ 10 mg/mL = 0.4 mL *Rationale: Concentration calculation. Always verify units cancel correctly*

Question 5: Step 1: 70 kg × 15 units/kg/hr = 1,050 units/hr Step 2: 25,000 units in 250 mL = 100 units/mL Step 3: 1,050 units/hr ÷ 100 units/mL = 10.5 mL/hr *Rationale: Weight-based dosing with concentration conversion*

Practice Exam 2: Clinical Integration

Question 6: A nurse is preparing insulin for a diabetic patient. The sliding scale orders 6 units of regular insulin subcutaneous for blood glucose 250 mg/dL. Available insulin is U-100. How many units should appear in the insulin syringe?

Question 7: A 5-year-old child weighing 18 kg has a fever and needs ibuprofen. The safe dose range is 5-10 mg/kg every 6 hours. What is the minimum and maximum safe dose for this child?

Question 8: A patient requires vancomycin 1 g IV over 60 minutes. The pharmacy provides vancomycin 1 g in 250 mL. Calculate the infusion pump rate in mL/hr.

Question 9: A premature infant weighing 2.2 pounds needs caffeine citrate 5 mg/kg IV. Available concentration is 20 mg/mL. Calculate the dose in mg and the volume in mL.

Question 10: A patient with heart failure receives furosemide 80 mg IV twice daily. Available vials contain 40 mg/4 mL. How many mL should the nurse administer per dose?

Solutions and Rationales:

Question 6: 6 units (no calculation needed with U-100 insulin and insulin syringe) *Rationale: U-100 insulin with insulin syringe reads directly in units*

Question 7: Minimum: 18 kg × 5 mg/kg = 90 mg per dose Maximum: 18 kg × 10 mg/kg = 180 mg per dose *Rationale: Safe dose range calculation using weight-based dosing*

Question 8: 250 mL ÷ 1 hour = 250 mL/hr *Rationale: Volume given over specified time equals pump rate*

Question 9: Step 1: Convert weight: 2.2 pounds ÷ 2.2 = 1 kg Step 2: Calculate dose: 1 kg × 5 mg/kg = 5 mg Step 3: Calculate volume: 5 mg ÷ 20 mg/mL = 0.25 mL *Rationale: Weight conversion required before weight-based calculation*

Question 10: 80 mg × (4 mL/40 mg) = 8 mL per dose *Rationale: Use available concentration to calculate volume needed*

Practice Exam 3: Advanced Applications

Question 11: A critical care patient weighing 75 kg requires dopamine at 10 mcg/kg/min. Available concentration is 400 mg in 250 mL. Calculate the infusion rate in mL/hr.

Question 12: A nurse is preparing to administer digoxin 0.25 mg PO daily. Available tablets are scored and contain 0.5 mg each. How many tablets should the nurse give?

Question 13: A patient needs potassium chloride 40 mEq added to 1,000 mL normal saline to infuse over 10 hours. What is the potassium concentration in mEq/L and the infusion rate in mL/hr?

Question 14: A 3-month-old infant weighing 5 kg needs acetaminophen 15 mg/kg every 6 hours. Available suspension contains 80 mg per 0.8 mL. Calculate the dose in mg and volume in mL.

Question 15: A patient receives regular insulin 10 units subcutaneous before meals. Available insulin pens deliver U-100 insulin. How should the nurse set the pen dial?

Solutions and Rationales:

Question 11: Step 1: 75 kg × 10 mcg/kg/min = 750 mcg/min = 45,000 mcg/hr Step 2: 400 mg in 250 mL = 1,600 mcg/mL
Step 3: 45,000 mcg/hr ÷ 1,600 mcg/mL = 28.1 mL/hr *Rationale: Weight-based dosing with time and concentration conversions*

Question 12: 0.25 mg ÷ 0.5 mg/tablet = 0.5 tablet (½ tablet) *Rationale: Tablet can be split because it's scored*

Question 13: Concentration: 40 mEq in 1,000 mL = 40 mEq/L Infusion rate: 1,000 mL ÷ 10 hours = 100 mL/hr *Rationale: Two separate calculations for concentration and rate*

Question 14: Dose: 5 kg × 15 mg/kg = 75 mg Volume: 75 mg × (0.8 mL/80 mg) = 0.75 mL *Rationale: Weight-based pediatric dosing with liquid calculation*

Question 15: Set pen dial to 10 units *Rationale: U-100 insulin pens calibrated to deliver units directly*

Competency Testing Throughout Career

Employment Competency Requirements

Healthcare employers require ongoing competency demonstration for medication administration, including:

Initial competency testing: Mathematical skills assessment during orientation **Annual competency verification**: Yearly testing to maintain medication administration privileges
High-alert medication competencies: Specialized testing for critical care drugs **Specialty area competencies**: Additional testing for specialized units (pediatrics, critical care, chemotherapy)

Competency Testing Strategies

Approach employment competency testing with the same systematic preparation used for NCLEX:

Review institutional policies: Learn facility-specific protocols and calculation methods **Practice with realistic scenarios**: Use clinical situations from your work environment **Maintain calculation fluency**: Practice regularly to keep skills sharp **Seek clarification**: Ask questions about policies or procedures before testing

Continuing Education and Skill Maintenance

Medication calculation skills require ongoing maintenance throughout your career:

Stay current with technology: Learn new pump systems and calculation software **Review complex cases**: Analyze difficult calculations from clinical practice **Attend continuing education**: Participate in medication safety and calculation updates **Mentor newer nurses**: Teaching calculations reinforces your own skills

Building Long-Term Competency

Systematic Skill Development

Your medication calculation journey extends far beyond initial competency testing. Build systematic approaches for lifelong learning:

Regular practice: Set aside time weekly for calculation practice **Real-world application**: Use every clinical calculation as a learning opportunity **Peer consultation**: Discuss complex calculations with colleagues **Professional development**: Pursue advanced certifications that require calculation competency

Technology Integration

Modern healthcare increasingly integrates technology with calculation skills:

Smart pump competency: Learn advanced pump features and safety systems **Electronic documentation**: Understand how calculations integrate with EHR systems **Mobile applications**: Use approved calculation apps while maintaining manual skills **Clinical decision support**: Leverage technology while maintaining independent calculation ability

Testing Success: Your Professional Foundation

NCLEX success and ongoing competency testing represent milestones in your professional development rather than endpoints. The calculation skills you master for these assessments become tools you use daily to protect patient safety and provide effective nursing care throughout your career.

Your systematic approach to calculation competency—built through progressive skill development, comprehensive practice, and confidence-building strategies—distinguishes you as a practitioner committed to mathematical precision and patient safety. These skills enable you to function confidently in any healthcare environment while maintaining the accuracy demanded by professional nursing practice.

The testing strategies and anxiety management techniques you develop serve you well beyond initial licensure, supporting continued professional growth and specialization throughout your nursing career. Each successful competency demonstration reinforces your commitment to excellence and your role as a trusted healthcare professional.

Your mastery of medication calculations, demonstrated through successful testing performance, opens doors to advanced practice opportunities while providing the foundation for safe, effective patient care in all your professional endeavors.

Key Learning Points

- NCLEX medication calculations integrate mathematical skills with clinical reasoning and nursing judgment
- Systematic test-taking strategies improve accuracy while managing examination anxiety and time pressure
- Progressive practice builds confidence through foundation skills to advanced clinical applications
- Competency testing continues throughout nursing careers, requiring ongoing skill maintenance and development

- Technology integration enhances calculation capabilities while maintaining the need for independent mathematical competency

Chapter 11: Dosage Calculations Practice Problems

Category 1: Basic Arithmetic & Fractions

Problem 1: Convert the fraction **3/4** to a decimal.
Solution:
Step 1: Divide numerator by denominator → 3 ÷ 4 = 0.75
Answer: 0.75
Explanation: Dividing numerator by denominator converts a fraction to decimal.

Problem 2: Convert the fraction **5/8** into a decimal number.
Solution:
Step 1: Divide numerator by denominator → 5 ÷ 8 = 0.625
Answer: 0.625
Explanation: Decimal equivalent found by division.

Problem 3: Add the fractions **2/5** and **1/10**. Express your answer as a simplified fraction.
Solution:
Step 1: Find the least common denominator (LCD) of 5 and 10, which is 10.
Step 2: Convert fractions: 2/5 = 4/10, 1/10 = 1/10
Step 3: Add numerators: 4 + 1 = 5
Step 4: Write sum over common denominator: 5/10
Step 5: Simplify fraction: 5/10 = 1/2
Answer: 1/2

Explanation: Convert to common denominator before adding fractions.

Problem 4: Subtract **3/7** from **5/7**. Write the answer as a fraction.
Solution:
Step 1: Since denominators are the same, subtract numerators: 5 - 3 = 2
Step 2: Write result over denominator: 2/7
Answer: 2/7
Explanation: Same denominator means subtract only numerators.

Problem 5: Multiply the fractions **2/3** by **3/4**. Simplify your answer.
Solution:
Step 1: Multiply numerators: $2 \times 3 = 6$
Step 2: Multiply denominators: $3 \times 4 = 12$
Step 3: Write fraction: 6/12
Step 4: Simplify fraction: 6/12 = 1/2
Answer: 1/2
Explanation: Multiply straight across numerator and denominator, then simplify.

Problem 6: Divide **4/5** by **2/3**. Express your answer as a simplified mixed number or fraction.
Solution:
Step 1: Division of fractions means multiply by reciprocal: $4/5 \div 2/3 = 4/5 \times 3/2$
Step 2: Multiply numerators: $4 \times 3 = 12$
Step 3: Multiply denominators: $5 \times 2 = 10$
Step 4: Write fraction: 12/10
Step 5: Simplify fraction: 12/10 = 6/5
Step 6: Convert to mixed number: 6/5 = 1 1/5
Answer: 1 1/5

Explanation: Multiply by reciprocal then simplify; convert improper fraction to mixed number.

Problem 7: Convert the decimal **0.2** to a simplified fraction.
Solution:
Step 1: Write decimal as fraction: $0.2 = 2/10$
Step 2: Simplify fraction: divide numerator and denominator by 2 →
$2/10 = 1/5$
Answer: 1/5
Explanation: Convert decimal to fraction and simplify.

Problem 8: Round the number **5.6789** to two decimal places.
Solution:
Step 1: Identify digit at hundredths place (second decimal place): 7
Step 2: Check the digit at the thousandths place (third decimal place):
8
Step 3: Since $8 \geq 5$, round the hundredths place up: 7 → 8
Step 4: Result: 5.68
Answer: 5.68
Explanation: Round up if next digit is 5 or greater.

Problem 9: Express **25%** as a decimal number.
Solution:
Step 1: Percent means per hundred → $25\% = 25/100$
Step 2: Divide 25 by $100 = 0.25$
Answer: 0.25
Explanation: Divide percentage by 100 to get decimal.

Problem 10: Calculate 15% of **200 mg**.
Solution:

Step 1: Convert percentage to decimal: 15% = 0.15
Step 2: Multiply decimal by total amount: 0.15 × 200 mg = 30 mg
Answer: 30 mg
Explanation: Convert percent to decimal and multiply.

Problem 11: Increase **90 mg** by one-third. Find the new amount.
Solution:
Step 1: Calculate one-third of 90 mg: 90 × (1/3) = 30 mg
Step 2: Add to original: 90 + 30 = 120 mg
Answer: 120 mg
Explanation: Find fraction of amount and add.

Problem 12: Decrease **250 mL** by 18%. What is the remaining volume?
Solution:
Step 1: Calculate percentage remaining: 100% - 18% = 82%
Step 2: Convert to decimal: 82% = 0.82
Step 3: Multiply: 0.82 × 250 mL = 205 mL
Answer: 205 mL
Explanation: Multiply original volume by remaining percent.

Problem 13: Convert the fraction ⅗ to a percentage.
Solution:
Step 1: Convert fraction to decimal: 3 ÷ 5 = 0.6
Step 2: Convert decimal to percent: 0.6 × 100 = 60%
Answer: 60%
Explanation: Decimal × 100 = percentage.

Problem 14: Express **2.4 g** as grams and milligrams.
Solution:

Step 1: Separate whole grams: 2 g
Step 2: Convert decimal part to mg: 0.4 g × 1000 = 400 mg
Answer: 2 g and 400 mg
Explanation: 1 g = 1000 mg.

Problem 15: Simplify the ratio **480 mg : 1.2 g** to the lowest terms using the same units.
Solution:
Step 1: Convert 1.2 g to mg: 1.2 × 1000 = 1200 mg
Step 2: Write ratio: 480 : 1200
Step 3: Divide both by 240: 480 ÷ 240 = 2, 1200 ÷ 240 = 5
Answer: 2 : 5
Explanation: Use same units; divide both by their greatest common factor.

Problem 16: Convert **0.028 kg** to milligrams.
Solution:
Step 1: Convert kg to g: 0.028 × 1000 = 28 g
Step 2: Convert g to mg: 28 × 1000 = 28000 mg
Answer: 28000 mg
Explanation: Multiply by 1000 twice (kg → g → mg).

Problem 17: Convert **65 μg** to milligrams.
Solution:
Step 1: 1 mg = 1000 μg
Step 2: Convert: 65 ÷ 1000 = 0.065 mg
Answer: 0.065 mg
Explanation: Divide micrograms by 1000.

Problem 18: A vial contains **0.75 g/3 mL**. Express the concentration in mg/mL.
Solution:
Step 1: Convert g to mg: 0.75 × 1000 = 750 mg
Step 2: Calculate concentration: 750 mg ÷ 3 mL = 250 mg/mL
Answer: 250 mg/mL
Explanation: Convert units and divide.

Problem 19: Convert **7.2 L** to millilitres.
Solution:
Step 1: 1 L = 1000 mL
Step 2: 7.2 × 1000 = 7200 mL
Answer: 7200 mL
Explanation: Multiply litres by 1000.

Problem 20: What percentage of a 500 mL bag is 125 mL?
Solution:
Step 1: Divide part by whole: 125 ÷ 500 = 0.25
Step 2: Convert to percentage: 0.25 × 100 = 25%
Answer: 25%
Explanation: Part/whole × 100 = percentage.

Problem 21: Find 10% of 450 mg.
Solution:
Step 1: Convert percentage to decimal: 10% = 0.10
Step 2: Multiply: 0.10 × 450 mg = 45 mg
Answer: 45 mg
Explanation: Multiply total by decimal equivalent of percent.

Problem 22: Add 3/8 and 1/4. Express answer as a simplified fraction.
Solution:
Step 1: Find LCD of 8 and 4 = 8
Step 2: Convert fractions: 3/8 = 3/8; 1/4 = 2/8
Step 3: Add numerators: 3 + 2 = 5
Step 4: Result: 5/8
Answer: 5/8
Explanation: Convert to common denominator before adding.

Problem 23: Multiply 7/9 by 3/5.
Solution:
Step 1: Multiply numerators: $7 \times 3 = 21$
Step 2: Multiply denominators: $9 \times 5 = 45$
Step 3: Simplify fraction: 21/45 = 7/15
Answer: 7/15
Explanation: Multiply straight across, then simplify.

Problem 24: Subtract 2/3 from 5/6.
Solution:
Step 1: Find LCD of 6 and 3 = 6
Step 2: Convert fractions: 5/6 = 5/6; 2/3 = 4/6
Step 3: Subtract numerators: 5 - 4 = 1
Step 4: Result: 1/6
Answer: 1/6
Explanation: Convert to common denominator, then subtract.

Problem 25: Convert 0.375 to a fraction in simplest form.
Solution:
Step 1: Write decimal as fraction: 375/1000
Step 2: Simplify by dividing numerator and denominator by 125: 375 ÷ 125 = 3; 1000 ÷ 125 = 8

Step 3: Result: 3/8
Answer: 3/8
Explanation: Convert decimal to fraction and simplify.

Problem 26: Round 24.678 to the nearest whole number.
Solution:
Step 1: Look at first decimal digit: 6 ($\geq$ 5)
Step 2: Round up: 24 $\rightarrow$ 25
Answer: 25
Explanation: Round up when digit right after decimal is 5 or more.

Problem 27: Convert 12.5% to a decimal.
Solution:
Step 1: Divide 12.5 by 100 = 0.125
Answer: 0.125
Explanation: Percent to decimal conversion.

Problem 28: Find 18% of 300 mL.
Solution:
Step 1: Convert percent to decimal: 18% = 0.18
Step 2: Multiply: 0.18 $\times$ 300 = 54 mL
Answer: 54 mL
Explanation: Multiply amount by decimal form of percentage.

Problem 29: Increase 120 mg by 25%.
Solution:
Step 1: Calculate 25% of 120 mg: 120 $\times$ 0.25 = 30 mg
Step 2: Add to original: 120 + 30 = 150 mg
Answer: 150 mg
Explanation: Add percent increase to original value.

Problem 30: Reduce 400 mL by 15%.
Solution:
Step 1: Calculate 15% of 400: $400 \times 0.15 = 60$ mL
Step 2: Subtract from original: 400 - 60 = 340 mL
Answer: 340 mL
Explanation: Subtract percent decrease from original value.

Category 2: Metric Conversions

Problem 51: Convert **0.5 grams** to milligrams.
Solution:
Step 1: 1 g = 1000 mg
Step 2: 0.5 × 1000 = 500 mg
Answer: 500 mg
Explanation: Multiply grams by 1000 to convert to milligrams.

Problem 52: Convert **750 mg** to grams.
Solution:
Step 1: 1 g = 1000 mg
Step 2: 750 ÷ 1000 = 0.75 g
Answer: 0.75 g
Explanation: Divide milligrams by 1000 to convert to grams.

Problem 53: Convert **3 liters** to milliliters.
Solution:
Step 1: 1 L = 1000 mL
Step 2: 3 × 1000 = 3000 mL
Answer: 3000 mL
Explanation: Multiply liters by 1000 to convert to milliliters.

Problem 54: Convert **2500 mL** to liters.
Solution:
Step 1: 1 L = 1000 mL
Step 2: 2500 ÷ 1000 = 2.5 L
Answer: 2.5 L
Explanation: Divide milliliters by 1000 to convert to liters.

Problem 55: Convert **120 micrograms (µg)** to milligrams (mg).
Solution:
Step 1: 1 mg = 1000 µg
Step 2: 120 ÷ 1000 = 0.12 mg
Answer: 0.12 mg
Explanation: Divide micrograms by 1000 to convert to milligrams.

Problem 56: Convert **2.5 mg** to micrograms (µg).
Solution:
Step 1: 1 mg = 1000 µg
Step 2: 2.5 × 1000 = 2500 µg
Answer: 2500 µg
Explanation: Multiply milligrams by 1000 to convert to micrograms.

Problem 57: Convert **0.25 kilograms (kg)** to grams (g).
Solution:
Step 1: 1 kg = 1000 g
Step 2: 0.25 × 1000 = 250 g
Answer: 250 g
Explanation: Multiply kilograms by 1000 to convert to grams.

Problem 58: Convert **3500 g** to kilograms (kg).
Solution:
Step 1: 1 kg = 1000 g
Step 2: 3500 ÷ 1000 = 3.5 kg
Answer: 3.5 kg
Explanation: Divide grams by 1000 to convert to kilograms.

Problem 59: Convert **0.4 milliliters (mL)** to microliters (μL).
Solution:
Step 1: 1 mL = 1000 μL
Step 2: 0.4 × 1000 = 400 μL
Answer: 400 μL
Explanation: Multiply milliliters by 1000 to convert to microliters.

Problem 60: Convert **4500 μL** to milliliters (mL).
Solution:
Step 1: 1 mL = 1000 μL
Step 2: 4500 ÷ 1000 = 4.5 mL
Answer: 4.5 mL
Explanation: Divide microliters by 1000 to convert to milliliters.

Problem 61: A medication vial contains **500 mg** of powder. How many grams does it contain?
Solution:
Step 1: 1 g = 1000 mg
Step 2: 500 ÷ 1000 = 0.5 g
Answer: 0.5 g
Explanation: Divide milligrams by 1000 to convert to grams.

Problem 62: Convert **0.0065 kg** to grams.
Solution:
Step 1: 1 kg = 1000 g
Step 2: 0.0065 × 1000 = 6.5 g
Answer: 6.5 g
Explanation: Multiply kilograms by 1000 to convert to grams.

Problem 63: Convert **15,000 micrograms (μg)** to milligrams (mg).
Solution:
Step 1: 1 mg = 1000 μg
Step 2: 15,000 ÷ 1000 = 15 mg
Answer: 15 mg
Explanation: Divide micrograms by 1000 to convert to milligrams.

Problem 64: Convert **0.025 L** to milliliters.
Solution:
Step 1: 1 L = 1000 mL
Step 2: 0.025 × 1000 = 25 mL
Answer: 25 mL
Explanation: Multiply liters by 1000 to convert to milliliters.

Problem 65: Convert **4.5 kg** to grams.
Solution:
Step 1: 1 kg = 1000 g
Step 2: 4.5 × 1000 = 4500 g
Answer: 4500 g
Explanation: Multiply kilograms by 1000 to convert to grams.

Problem 66: A prescription is for **0.75 g** of medication. How many milligrams should be given?
Solution:
Step 1: 1 g = 1000 mg
Step 2: 0.75 × 1000 = 750 mg
Answer: 750 mg
Explanation: Multiply grams by 1000.

Problem 67: Convert **0.02 mg** to micrograms.
Solution:
Step 1: 1 mg = 1000 µg
Step 2: 0.02 × 1000 = 20 µg
Answer: 20 µg
Explanation: Multiply milligrams by 1000.

Problem 68: Convert **1000 mL** to liters.
Solution:
Step 1: 1 L = 1000 mL
Step 2: 1000 ÷ 1000 = 1 L
Answer: 1 L
Explanation: Divide milliliters by 1000.

Problem 69: Convert **3.6 L** to milliliters.
Solution:
Step 1: 1 L = 1000 mL
Step 2: 3.6 × 1000 = 3600 mL
Answer: 3600 mL
Explanation: Multiply liters by 1000.

Problem 70: A vial contains **1.5 g** of drug powder. How many milligrams is this?
Solution:
Step 1: 1 g = 1000 mg
Step 2: 1.5 × 1000 = 1500 mg
Answer: 1500 mg
Explanation: Multiply grams by 1000.

Problem 71: Convert **0.0035 kg** to grams.
Solution:
Step 1: 1 kg = 1000 g
Step 2: 0.0035 × 1000 = 3.5 g
Answer: 3.5 g
Explanation: Multiply kilograms by 1000.

Problem 72: Convert **2500 micrograms (µg)** to milligrams (mg).
Solution:
Step 1: 1 mg = 1000 µg
Step 2: 2500 ÷ 1000 = 2.5 mg
Answer: 2.5 mg
Explanation: Divide micrograms by 1000.

Problem 73: Convert **0.5 mL** to microliters (µL).
Solution:
Step 1: 1 mL = 1000 µL
Step 2: 0.5 × 1000 = 500 µL
Answer: 500 µL
Explanation: Multiply milliliters by 1000.

Problem 74: Convert **12,000 µL** to milliliters (mL).
Solution:
Step 1: 1 mL = 1000 µL
Step 2: 12,000 ÷ 1000 = 12 mL
Answer: 12 mL
Explanation: Divide microliters by 1000.

Problem 75: Convert **3.75 g** to milligrams (mg).
Solution:

Step 1: 1 g = 1000 mg
Step 2: 3.75 × 1000 = 3750 mg
Answer: 3750 mg
Explanation: Multiply grams by 1000.

Problem 76: Convert **4000 mg** to grams (g).
Solution:
Step 1: 1 g = 1000 mg
Step 2: 4000 ÷ 1000 = 4 g
Answer: 4 g
Explanation: Divide milligrams by 1000.

Problem 77: Convert **0.09 L** to milliliters (mL).
Solution:
Step 1: 1 L = 1000 mL
Step 2: 0.09 × 1000 = 90 mL
Answer: 90 mL
Explanation: Multiply liters by 1000.

Problem 78: Convert **650 mL** to liters (L).
Solution:
Step 1: 1 L = 1000 mL
Step 2: 650 ÷ 1000 = 0.65 L
Answer: 0.65 L
Explanation: Divide milliliters by 1000.

Problem 79: Convert **0.0005 kg** to grams (g).
Solution:
Step 1: 1 kg = 1000 g
Step 2: 0.0005 × 1000 = 0.5 g

Answer: 0.5 g
Explanation: Multiply kilograms by 1000.

Problem 80: Convert **0.002 L** to milliliters (mL).
Solution:
Step 1: 1 L = 1000 mL
Step 2: 0.002 × 1000 = 2 mL
Answer: 2 mL
Explanation: Multiply liters by 1000.

Problem 81: Convert **150 µg** to milligrams (mg).
Solution:
Step 1: 1 mg = 1000 µg
Step 2: 150 ÷ 1000 = 0.15 mg
Answer: 0.15 mg
Explanation: Divide micrograms by 1000.

Problem 82: Convert **5 mg** to micrograms (µg).
Solution:
Step 1: 1 mg = 1000 µg
Step 2: 5 × 1000 = 5000 µg
Answer: 5000 µg
Explanation: Multiply milligrams by 1000.

Problem 83: Convert **0.025 kg** to grams (g).
Solution:
Step 1: 1 kg = 1000 g
Step 2: 0.025 × 1000 = 25 g
Answer: 25 g
Explanation: Multiply kilograms by 1000.

Problem 84: Convert **1200 g** to kilograms (kg).
Solution:
Step 1: 1 kg = 1000 g
Step 2: 1200 ÷ 1000 = 1.2 kg
Answer: 1.2 kg
Explanation: Divide grams by 1000.

Problem 85: Convert **0.01 L** to milliliters (mL).
Solution:
Step 1: 1 L = 1000 mL
Step 2: 0.01 × 1000 = 10 mL
Answer: 10 mL
Explanation: Multiply liters by 1000.

Problem 86: Convert **850 mL** to liters (L).
Solution:
Step 1: 1 L = 1000 mL
Step 2: 850 ÷ 1000 = 0.85 L
Answer: 0.85 L
Explanation: Divide milliliters by 1000.

Problem 87: Convert **0.6 g** to milligrams (mg).
Solution:
Step 1: 1 g = 1000 mg
Step 2: 0.6 × 1000 = 600 mg
Answer: 600 mg
Explanation: Multiply grams by 1000.

Problem 88: Convert **1250 mg** to grams (g).
Solution:
Step 1: 1 g = 1000 mg
Step 2: 1250 ÷ 1000 = 1.25 g
Answer: 1.25 g
Explanation: Divide milligrams by 1000.

Problem 89: Convert **0.0045 L** to milliliters (mL).
Solution:
Step 1: 1 L = 1000 mL
Step 2: 0.0045 × 1000 = 4.5 mL
Answer: 4.5 mL
Explanation: Multiply liters by 1000.

Problem 90: Convert **750 mL** to liters (L).
Solution:
Step 1: 1 L = 1000 mL
Step 2: 750 ÷ 1000 = 0.75 L
Answer: 0.75 L
Explanation: Divide milliliters by 1000.

Problem 91: Convert **0.0009 kg** to grams (g).
Solution:
Step 1: 1 kg = 1000 g
Step 2: 0.0009 × 1000 = 0.9 g
Answer: 0.9 g
Explanation: Multiply kilograms by 1000.

Problem 92: Convert **1800 µg** to milligrams (mg).
Solution:

Step 1: 1 mg = 1000 µg
Step 2: 1800 ÷ 1000 = 1.8 mg
Answer: 1.8 mg
Explanation: Divide micrograms by 1000.

Problem 93: Convert **0.35 mL** to microliters (µL).
Solution:
Step 1: 1 mL = 1000 µL
Step 2: 0.35 × 1000 = 350 µL
Answer: 350 µL
Explanation: Multiply milliliters by 1000.

Problem 94: Convert **6000 µL** to milliliters (mL).
Solution:
Step 1: 1 mL = 1000 µL
Step 2: 6000 ÷ 1000 = 6 mL
Answer: 6 mL
Explanation: Divide microliters by 1000.

Problem 95: Convert **2.1 g** to milligrams (mg).
Solution:
Step 1: 1 g = 1000 mg
Step 2: 2.1 × 1000 = 2100 mg
Answer: 2100 mg
Explanation: Multiply grams by 1000.

Problem 96: Convert **5000 mg** to grams (g).
Solution:
Step 1: 1 g = 1000 mg
Step 2: 5000 ÷ 1000 = 5 g

Answer: 5 g
Explanation: Divide milligrams by 1000.

Problem 97: Convert **0.007 L** to milliliters (mL).
Solution:
Step 1: 1 L = 1000 mL
Step 2: 0.007 × 1000 = 7 mL
Answer: 7 mL
Explanation: Multiply liters by 1000.

Problem 98: Convert **920 mL** to liters (L).
Solution:
Step 1: 1 L = 1000 mL
Step 2: 920 ÷ 1000 = 0.92 L
Answer: 0.92 L
Explanation: Divide milliliters by 1000.

Problem 99: Convert **0.8 g** to milligrams (mg).
Solution:
Step 1: 1 g = 1000 mg
Step 2: 0.8 × 1000 = 800 mg
Answer: 800 mg
Explanation: Multiply grams by 1000.

Problem 100: Convert **2750 mg** to grams (g).
Solution:
Step 1: 1 g = 1000 mg
Step 2: 2750 ÷ 1000 = 2.75 g
Answer: 2.75 g
Explanation: Divide milligrams by 1000.

Category 3: Ratio & Proportion

Problem 101: A medication contains 100 mg in 2 mL. How many milliliters contain 150 mg?
Solution:
Step 1: Set up proportion: 100 mg : 2 mL = 150 mg : x mL
Step 2: Cross multiply: 100 × x = 150 × 2
Step 3: Solve for x: x = (150 × 2) ÷ 100 = 300 ÷ 100 = 3 mL
Answer: 3 mL
Explanation: Use cross multiplication to solve proportion.

Problem 102: A medication has a concentration of 250 mg/5 mL. How many milliliters are needed for a 500 mg dose?
Solution:
Step 1: Set proportion: 250 mg : 5 mL = 500 mg : x mL
Step 2: Cross multiply: 250 × x = 500 × 5
Step 3: Solve for x: x = (500 × 5) ÷ 250 = 2500 ÷ 250 = 10 mL
Answer: 10 mL
Explanation: Cross multiplication to find volume for desired dose.

Problem 103: If 1 part medication is mixed with 3 parts diluent, what is the concentration ratio of medication to total solution?
Solution:
Step 1: Total parts = 1 (medication) + 3 (diluent) = 4 parts
Step 2: Medication fraction = 1 part medication ÷ 4 total parts = 1/4
Step 3: Ratio is medication : total = 1 : 4
Answer: 1:4
Explanation: Ratio of medication to total volume.

Problem 104: A tablet contains 150 mg of active drug. If 3 tablets are given, how much drug is administered?
Solution:
Step 1: Multiply: 150 mg × 3 tablets = 450 mg
Answer: 450 mg
Explanation: Multiply dose per tablet by number of tablets.

Problem 105: You need to administer 120 mg of a drug. Each tablet contains 80 mg. How many tablets do you need?
Solution:
Step 1: Divide required dose by tablet strength: 120 mg ÷ 80 mg/tablet = 1.5 tablets
Answer: 1.5 tablets
Explanation: Divide dose by strength to find number of tablets.

Problem 106: A liquid medication is labeled as 60 mg per 5 mL. How many milliliters deliver 90 mg?
Solution:
Step 1: Set proportion: 60 mg : 5 mL = 90 mg : x mL
Step 2: Cross multiply: 60 × x = 90 × 5
Step 3: Solve: x = 450 ÷ 60 = 7.5 mL
Answer: 7.5 mL
Explanation: Use ratio to find volume for given dose.

Problem 107: If a solution contains 500 mg of drug in 50 mL, what is the concentration in mg/mL?
Solution:
Step 1: Divide total drug by total volume: 500 mg ÷ 50 mL = 10 mg/mL
Answer: 10 mg/mL
Explanation: Concentration equals amount per volume.

136

Problem 108: How many milliliters of a 20 mg/mL solution are needed to deliver a 50 mg dose?
Solution:
Step 1: Use formula: Volume (mL) = Dose (mg) ÷ Concentration (mg/mL)
Step 2: Volume = 50 mg ÷ 20 mg/mL = 2.5 mL
Answer: 2.5 mL
Explanation: Dose divided by concentration.

Problem 109: You have a 10% solution and want to make 500 mL of a 4% solution by dilution. How much stock solution and diluent will you use?
Solution:
Step 1: Use alligation:

- Parts of stock: (10 - 4) = 6
- Parts of diluent: (4 - 0) = 4
  Step 2: Total parts = 6 + 4 = 10 parts
  Step 3: Volume of stock: (6/10) × 500 = 300 mL
  Step 4: Volume of diluent: 500 - 300 = 200 mL
  Answer: 300 mL stock, 200 mL diluent
  Explanation: Alligation method to mix solutions.

Problem 110: A 1:5 dilution is prepared. If the final volume is 60 mL, how much of the stock solution is used?
Solution:
Step 1: Ratio 1:5 means 1 part stock + 5 parts diluent = 6 parts total
Step 2: Volume of stock = (1/6) × 60 = 10 mL
Answer: 10 mL
Explanation: Divide total volume by sum of parts, multiply by stock parts.

Problem 111: A patient is prescribed 18 mg of medication. The vial concentration is 6 mg/mL. How many milliliters should be administered?
Solution:
Step 1: Volume = Dose ÷ Concentration = 18 mg ÷ 6 mg/mL = 3 mL
Answer: 3 mL
Explanation: Dose divided by concentration gives volume.

Problem 112: A syrup contains 150 mg in 5 mL. How much syrup is required to provide 225 mg?
Solution:
Step 1: Set proportion: 150 mg : 5 mL = 225 mg : x mL
Step 2: Cross multiply: 150 × x = 225 × 5
Step 3: Solve for x: x = 1125 ÷ 150 = 7.5 mL
Answer: 7.5 mL
Explanation: Use ratio for volume.

Problem 113: A medication requires 40 mg every 6 hours. How many milligrams will be administered in 24 hours?
Solution:
Step 1: Number of doses in 24 hours: 24 ÷ 6 = 4
Step 2: Total dose: 40 mg × 4 = 160 mg
Answer: 160 mg
Explanation: Multiply dose per administration by number of doses.

Problem 114: The doctor orders 300 mg of medication. You have 250 mg tablets. How many tablets do you give?
Solution:
Step 1: Tablets = 300 mg ÷ 250 mg/tablet = 1.2 tablets

Answer: 1.2 tablets
Explanation: Divide ordered dose by tablet strength.

Problem 115: A drug is supplied as 500 mg in 5 mL. How many milliliters will provide 750 mg?
Solution:
Step 1: Set proportion: 500 mg : 5 mL = 750 mg : x mL
Step 2: Cross multiply: 500 × x = 750 × 5
Step 3: Solve: x = 3750 ÷ 500 = 7.5 mL
Answer: 7.5 mL
Explanation: Use cross multiplication.

Problem 116: How many milliliters of a 50 mg/mL solution are needed to provide 200 mg?
Solution:
Step 1: Volume = Dose ÷ Concentration = 200 mg ÷ 50 mg/mL = 4 mL
Answer: 4 mL
Explanation: Divide dose by concentration.

Problem 117: A child needs 25 mg of medicine. The syrup contains 5 mg per teaspoon (5 mL). How many teaspoons will you give?
Solution:
Step 1: Volume in mL = Dose ÷ Concentration = 25 mg ÷ (5 mg/5 mL) = 25 mg ÷ 1 mg/mL = 25 mL
Step 2: Teaspoons = 25 mL ÷ 5 mL/teaspoon = 5 teaspoons
Answer: 5 teaspoons
Explanation: Calculate total mL, convert to teaspoons.

Problem 118: How many tablets are required if the order is 150 mg and tablets contain 75 mg each?
Solution:
Step 1: Tablets = 150 mg ÷ 75 mg/tablet = 2 tablets
Answer: 2 tablets
Explanation: Divide ordered dose by tablet strength.

Problem 119: A medication dose is 2 mg/kg/day in divided doses every 8 hours. Patient weighs 30 kg. What is the dose per administration?
Solution:
Step 1: Total daily dose = 2 mg/kg × 30 kg = 60 mg/day
Step 2: Number of doses per day = 24 ÷ 8 = 3 doses
Step 3: Dose per administration = 60 mg ÷ 3 = 20 mg
Answer: 20 mg per dose every 8 hours
Explanation: Calculate total daily dose, divide by number of doses.

Problem 120: You have a 10 mg/mL concentration and need to administer 35 mg. How many milliliters will you give?
Solution:
Step 1: Volume = Dose ÷ Concentration = 35 mg ÷ 10 mg/mL = 3.5 mL
Answer: 3.5 mL
Explanation: Dose divided by concentration.

Problem 121: A solution is labeled 500 mg/10 mL. How much solution will provide 250 mg?
Solution:
Step 1: Set proportion: 500 mg : 10 mL = 250 mg : x mL
Step 2: Cross multiply: 500 × x = 250 × 10
Step 3: Solve: x = 2500 ÷ 500 = 5 mL

Answer: 5 mL
Explanation: Use ratio to find volume.

Problem 122: A doctor orders 750 mg of a drug. The vial concentration is 250 mg/mL. How many milliliters are required?
Solution:
Step 1: Volume = Dose ÷ Concentration = 750 mg ÷ 250 mg/mL = 3 mL
Answer: 3 mL
Explanation: Dose divided by concentration.

Problem 123: How many tablets do you need if the order is 500 mg and tablets contain 125 mg?
Solution:
Step 1: Tablets = 500 mg ÷ 125 mg/tablet = 4 tablets
Answer: 4 tablets
Explanation: Divide ordered dose by tablet strength.

Problem 124: A solution contains 400 mg in 16 mL. What is the concentration in mg/mL?
Solution:
Step 1: Concentration = 400 mg ÷ 16 mL = 25 mg/mL
Answer: 25 mg/mL
Explanation: Divide amount by volume.

Problem 125: You have a stock solution of 50 mg/mL. How many milliliters deliver 200 mg?
Solution:
Step 1: Volume = Dose ÷ Concentration = 200 mg ÷ 50 mg/mL = 4 mL

Answer: 4 mL
Explanation: Dose divided by concentration.

Problem 126: A medication label shows 400 mg in 20 mL. How many milliliters provide 100 mg?
Solution:
Step 1: Set proportion: 400 mg : 20 mL = 100 mg : x mL
Step 2: Cross multiply: $400 \times x = 100 \times 20$
Step 3: Solve: x = 2000 ÷ 400 = 5 mL
Answer: 5 mL
Explanation: Cross multiplication to find unknown volume.

Problem 127: You have a solution of 75 mg/3 mL. How many milliliters are needed for a 150 mg dose?
Solution:
Step 1: Set proportion: 75 mg : 3 mL = 150 mg : x mL
Step 2: Cross multiply: $75 \times x = 150 \times 3$
Step 3: Solve: x = 450 ÷ 75 = 6 mL
Answer: 6 mL
Explanation: Use proportion to calculate volume.

Problem 128: A drug is supplied as 500 mg in 50 mL. How many milliliters contain 200 mg?
Solution:
Step 1: Set proportion: 500 mg : 50 mL = 200 mg : x mL
Step 2: Cross multiply: $500 \times x = 200 \times 50$
Step 3: Solve: x = 10,000 ÷ 500 = 20 mL
Answer: 20 mL
Explanation: Proportion calculation for volume.

Problem 129: A vial has 300 mg of drug in 30 mL. How much volume contains 100 mg?
Solution:
Step 1: Set proportion: 300 mg : 30 mL = 100 mg : x mL
Step 2: Cross multiply: 300 × x = 100 × 30
Step 3: Solve: x = 3000 ÷ 300 = 10 mL
Answer: 10 mL
Explanation: Use ratio and proportion.

Problem 130: The doctor orders 250 mg of medication. You have 125 mg tablets. How many tablets do you administer?
Solution:
Step 1: Tablets = 250 mg ÷ 125 mg/tablet = 2 tablets
Answer: 2 tablets
Explanation: Divide dose by tablet strength.

Problem 131: A medication is available as 200 mg per 10 mL. How many milliliters provide 400 mg?
Solution:
Step 1: Set proportion: 200 mg : 10 mL = 400 mg : x mL
Step 2: Cross multiply: 200 × x = 400 × 10
Step 3: Solve: x = 4000 ÷ 200 = 20 mL
Answer: 20 mL
Explanation: Proportional relationship to find volume.

Problem 132: A patient requires 100 mg of medication. The concentration is 50 mg/mL. How many milliliters should be administered?
Solution:
Step 1: Volume = Dose ÷ Concentration = 100 mg ÷ 50 mg/mL = 2 mL

Answer: 2 mL
Explanation: Divide dose by concentration.

Problem 133: You need to prepare 500 mL of a 5% solution by diluting a 10% stock solution. How much stock and diluent do you need?
Solution:
Step 1: Use alligation:

- Parts stock = 10 - 5 = 5
- Parts diluent = 5 - 0 = 5
  Step 2: Total parts = 5 + 5 = 10
  Step 3: Volume of stock = (5/10) × 500 = 250 mL
  Step 4: Volume of diluent = 500 - 250 = 250 mL
  Answer: 250 mL stock and 250 mL diluent
  Explanation: Use alligation for dilution.

Problem 134: A 1:4 mixture requires 20 mL total volume. How much of the stock solution is needed?
Solution:
Step 1: Ratio total parts = 1 + 4 = 5
Step 2: Volume stock = (1/5) × 20 = 4 mL
Answer: 4 mL
Explanation: Calculate portion of total volume.

Problem 135: A solution contains 150 mg in 10 mL. How much volume will provide 75 mg?
Solution:
Step 1: Set proportion: 150 mg : 10 mL = 75 mg : x mL
Step 2: Cross multiply: 150 × x = 75 × 10
Step 3: Solve: x = 750 ÷ 150 = 5 mL

Answer: 5 mL
Explanation: Use ratio to find volume.

Problem 136: The doctor orders 600 mg of a drug. The medication is supplied as 300 mg tablets. How many tablets should be given?
Solution:
Step 1: Tablets = 600 mg ÷ 300 mg/tablet = 2 tablets
Answer: 2 tablets
Explanation: Divide ordered dose by tablet strength.

Problem 137: A medication is supplied as 20 mg/mL. How many milliliters provide 80 mg?
Solution:
Step 1: Volume = Dose ÷ Concentration = 80 mg ÷ 20 mg/mL = 4 mL
Answer: 4 mL
Explanation: Divide dose by concentration.

Problem 138: A child weighs 15 kg and is prescribed 10 mg/kg/day of medication divided into 3 doses. How much is each dose?
Solution:
Step 1: Total daily dose = 10 mg/kg × 15 kg = 150 mg
Step 2: Dose per administration = 150 mg ÷ 3 = 50 mg
Answer: 50 mg per dose
Explanation: Multiply weight by dose and divide by doses.

Problem 139: A medication label reads 500 mg in 25 mL. How many milliliters provide 250 mg?
Solution:
Step 1: Set proportion: 500 mg : 25 mL = 250 mg : x mL
Step 2: Cross multiply: 500 × x = 250 × 25

Step 3: Solve: x = 6250 ÷ 500 = 12.5 mL
Answer: 12.5 mL
Explanation: Use proportion to calculate volume.

Problem 140: You have 75 mg tablets. How many tablets are needed for a 300 mg dose?
Solution:
Step 1: Tablets = 300 mg ÷ 75 mg/tablet = 4 tablets
Answer: 4 tablets
Explanation: Divide dose by tablet strength.

Problem 141: A medication concentration is 100 mg/4 mL. How many milliliters are required for a 50 mg dose?
Solution:
Step 1: Set proportion: 100 mg : 4 mL = 50 mg : x mL
Step 2: Cross multiply: $100 \times x = 50 \times 4$
Step 3: Solve: x = 200 ÷ 100 = 2 mL
Answer: 2 mL
Explanation: Use ratio to find volume.

Problem 142: A patient requires 120 mg of medication. The vial contains 60 mg/mL. How many milliliters should be administered?
Solution:
Step 1: Volume = Dose ÷ Concentration = 120 mg ÷ 60 mg/mL = 2 mL
Answer: 2 mL
Explanation: Divide dose by concentration.

Problem 143: The order is 250 mg of medication. Tablets contain 125 mg each. How many tablets do you administer?

Solution:
Step 1: Tablets = 250 mg ÷ 125 mg/tablet = 2 tablets
Answer: 2 tablets
Explanation: Divide ordered dose by tablet strength.

Problem 144: A medication concentration is 30 mg/mL. How many milliliters provide 90 mg?
Solution:
Step 1: Volume = Dose ÷ Concentration = 90 mg ÷ 30 mg/mL = 3 mL
Answer: 3 mL
Explanation: Divide dose by concentration.

Problem 145: A medication is ordered at 0.5 mg/kg for a 60 kg patient. How much medication is ordered?
Solution:
Step 1: Dose = 0.5 mg/kg × 60 kg = 30 mg
Answer: 30 mg
Explanation: Multiply weight by dose per kg.

Problem 146: How many tablets are needed if the order is 375 mg and tablets contain 125 mg?
Solution:
Step 1: Tablets = 375 mg ÷ 125 mg/tablet = 3 tablets
Answer: 3 tablets
Explanation: Divide dose by tablet strength.

Problem 147: A solution contains 40 mg/mL. How many milliliters deliver 100 mg?
Solution:
Step 1: Volume = Dose ÷ Concentration = 100 mg ÷ 40 mg/mL = 2.5

mL
Answer: 2.5 mL
Explanation: Divide dose by concentration.

Problem 148: The patient requires 180 mg of medication. The concentration is 90 mg per 5 mL. How many milliliters do you administer?
Solution:
Step 1: Set proportion: 90 mg : 5 mL = 180 mg : x mL
Step 2: Cross multiply: $90 \times x = 180 \times 5$
Step 3: Solve: $x = 900 \div 90 = 10$ mL
Answer: 10 mL
Explanation: Use proportion to calculate volume.

Problem 149: A medication contains 50 mg/mL. How many milliliters provide 125 mg?
Solution:
Step 1: Volume = Dose ÷ Concentration = 125 mg ÷ 50 mg/mL = 2.5 mL
Answer: 2.5 mL
Explanation: Divide dose by concentration.

Problem 150: The doctor orders 350 mg of medication. The tablets contain 175 mg. How many tablets are required?
Solution:
Step 1: Tablets = 350 mg ÷ 175 mg/tablet = 2 tablets
Answer: 2 tablets
Explanation: Divide dose by tablet strength.

Category 4: Body Weight-Based Dosing

Problem 151: A doctor orders 10 mg/kg/day of medication divided into two equal doses for a patient weighing 70 kg. What is the dose per administration?
Solution:
Step 1: Calculate total daily dose: 10 mg/kg × 70 kg = 700 mg/day
Step 2: Divide total daily dose by number of doses: 700 mg ÷ 2 = 350 mg per dose
Answer: 350 mg per dose
Explanation: Multiply weight by dose per kg, then divide by doses per day.

Problem 152: A medication is ordered at 5 mg/kg every 8 hours. Patient weighs 50 kg. How much medication is given per dose?
Solution:
Step 1: Calculate dose per administration: 5 mg/kg × 50 kg = 250 mg per dose
Answer: 250 mg every 8 hours
Explanation: Multiply weight by dose per kg.

Problem 153: A child weighs 20 kg and is prescribed 15 mg/kg/day of a drug. What is the total daily dose?
Solution:
Step 1: Multiply weight by dose per kg: 20 kg × 15 mg/kg = 300 mg/day
Answer: 300 mg per day
Explanation: Multiply weight by daily dose per kg.

Problem 154: A patient weighs 65 kg and requires a dose of 7 mg/kg/day divided into three doses. What is the amount per dose?
Solution:
Step 1: Calculate total daily dose: 7 mg/kg × 65 kg = 455 mg/day
Step 2: Divide by 3 doses: 455 mg ÷ 3 = approximately 151.7 mg per dose
Answer: 151.7 mg per dose
Explanation: Multiply weight by dose, divide by number of doses.

Problem 155: A medication is ordered at 4 mg/kg every 12 hours for a 30 kg child. How many milligrams per dose?
Solution:
Step 1: Calculate dose: 4 mg/kg × 30 kg = 120 mg per dose
Answer: 120 mg every 12 hours
Explanation: Multiply weight by mg/kg dose.

Problem 156: Patient weighs 45 kg and is ordered 250 mg of medication. Is the dose within the recommended 5 mg/kg?
Solution:
Step 1: Calculate maximum recommended dose: 5 mg/kg × 45 kg = 225 mg
Step 2: Compare ordered dose: 250 mg > 225 mg (overdose)
Answer: No, dose exceeds recommended 5 mg/kg limit
Explanation: Calculate recommended dose and compare.

Problem 157: A child weighs 18 kg. The order is 10 mg/kg/day given in 4 doses. What is the dose per administration?
Solution:
Step 1: Total daily dose = 10 mg/kg × 18 kg = 180 mg/day
Step 2: Divide by 4 doses: 180 mg ÷ 4 = 45 mg per dose
Answer: 45 mg every 6 hours
Explanation: Multiply weight by dose and divide by frequency.

Problem 158: A patient weighing 70 kg is ordered a medication at 6 mg/kg/day in 3 divided doses. Calculate the dose per administration.
Solution:
Step 1: Calculate total daily dose: 6 mg/kg × 70 kg = 420 mg/day
Step 2: Divide by 3 doses: 420 mg ÷ 3 = 140 mg per dose
Answer: 140 mg per dose
Explanation: Multiply weight by dose, divide by doses per day.

Problem 159: An order calls for 8 mg/kg/day for a 55 kg patient, given in two doses. What is the dose per administration?
Solution:
Step 1: Total daily dose: 8 mg/kg × 55 kg = 440 mg/day
Step 2: Dose per administration: 440 mg ÷ 2 = 220 mg
Answer: 220 mg every 12 hours
Explanation: Multiply weight by dose and divide by doses.

Problem 160: The recommended dose is 0.1 mg/kg/day. How much will a 25 kg patient receive per day?
Solution:
Step 1: Calculate total dose: 0.1 mg/kg × 25 kg = 2.5 mg/day
Answer: 2.5 mg per day
Explanation: Multiply weight by dose per kg.

Problem 161: A child weighs 15 kg and needs 15 mg/kg/day divided into three doses. How many milligrams per dose?
Solution:
Step 1: Total daily dose: 15 mg/kg × 15 kg = 225 mg/day
Step 2: Divide by 3 doses: 225 mg ÷ 3 = 75 mg per dose
Answer: 75 mg every 8 hours
Explanation: Multiply weight by dose, divide by frequency.

Problem 162: A 60 kg adult requires 500 mg of medication per day. What is the dose in mg/kg?
Solution:
Step 1: Dose per kg: 500 mg ÷ 60 kg = 8.33 mg/kg/day
Answer: 8.33 mg/kg/day
Explanation: Divide dose by patient weight.

Problem 163: Calculate the dose per administration for a 40 kg patient prescribed 12 mg/kg/day divided into 4 doses.
Solution:
Step 1: Total daily dose = 12 mg/kg × 40 kg = 480 mg/day
Step 2: Dose per administration = 480 mg ÷ 4 = 120 mg per dose
Answer: 120 mg every 6 hours
Explanation: Multiply weight by dose, divide by doses.

Problem 164: An order is 20 mg/kg/day for a patient weighing 8 kg. How much medication will be given daily?
Solution:
Step 1: Calculate total dose: 20 mg/kg × 8 kg = 160 mg/day
Answer: 160 mg per day
Explanation: Multiply dose per kg by weight.

Problem 165: A patient weighs 28 kg and is prescribed 1.5 mg/kg every 8 hours. What is the dose per administration?
Solution:
Step 1: Calculate per dose: 1.5 mg/kg × 28 kg = 42 mg
Answer: 42 mg every 8 hours
Explanation: Multiply weight by mg/kg dose.

Problem 166: Calculate the total daily dose for a 45 kg patient prescribed 25 mg/kg/day.
Solution:
Step 1: Multiply dose per kg by weight: 25 mg/kg × 45 kg = 1125 mg/day
Answer: 1125 mg per day
Explanation: Multiply weight by dose.

Problem 167: A drug is ordered at 0.5 mg/kg/day for a patient weighing 18 kg. How much medication is needed per day?
Solution:
Step 1: Calculate: 0.5 mg/kg × 18 kg = 9 mg/day
Answer: 9 mg per day
Explanation: Multiply weight by dose.

Problem 168: How many milligrams per dose will a 70 kg patient receive if prescribed 60 mg/kg/day in three doses?
Solution:
Step 1: Total daily dose: 60 mg/kg × 70 kg = 4200 mg/day
Step 2: Dose per administration: 4200 mg ÷ 3 = 1400 mg
Answer: 1400 mg per dose
Explanation: Multiply weight by dose, divide by number of doses.

Problem 169: A patient weighs 55 kg. Order is 8 mg/kg/day divided into two doses. What is the dose per administration?
Solution:
Step 1: Total dose: 8 mg/kg × 55 kg = 440 mg
Step 2: Dose per administration: 440 ÷ 2 = 220 mg
Answer: 220 mg every 12 hours
Explanation: Multiply weight by dose, divide by doses.

Problem 170: A pediatric patient weighs 22 kg and is prescribed 20 mg/kg/day divided into four doses. What is the dose per administration?
Solution:
Step 1: Total daily dose = 20 mg/kg × 22 kg = 440 mg
Step 2: Dose per administration = 440 mg ÷ 4 = 110 mg
Answer: 110 mg every 6 hours
Explanation: Multiply weight by dose, divide by frequency.

Problem 171: A patient weighing 10 kg needs 2.5 mg/kg/day of medication. Calculate total daily dose.
Solution:
Step 1: Multiply weight by dose: 2.5 mg/kg × 10 kg = 25 mg
Answer: 25 mg per day
Explanation: Multiply weight by dose.

Problem 172: A medication order calls for 3 mg/kg/day for a 40 kg patient given in two doses. Find dose per administration.
Solution:
Step 1: Total daily dose = 3 mg/kg × 40 kg = 120 mg
Step 2: Divide by 2: 120 mg ÷ 2 = 60 mg
Answer: 60 mg every 12 hours
Explanation: Multiply weight by dose, divide by doses.

Problem 173: Calculate the dose per administration for a patient weighing 50 kg prescribed 1.2 mg/kg/day divided into three doses.
Solution:
Step 1: Total daily dose = 1.2 mg/kg × 50 kg = 60 mg
Step 2: Divide by 3 doses: 60 mg ÷ 3 = 20 mg per dose
Answer: 20 mg every 8 hours
Explanation: Multiply weight by dose, divide by doses.

Problem 174: A child weighs 12 kg and is ordered 10 mg/kg/day divided into two doses. What is the dose per administration?
Solution:
Step 1: Total daily dose = 10 mg/kg × 12 kg = 120 mg
Step 2: Divide by 2 doses: 120 mg ÷ 2 = 60 mg
Answer: 60 mg every 12 hours
Explanation: Multiply weight by dose, divide by doses.

Problem 175: A medication is prescribed as 7 mg/kg/day for a patient weighing 38 kg, divided into four doses. What is the dose per administration?
Solution:
Step 1: Total dose = 7 mg/kg × 38 kg = 266 mg
Step 2: Dose per administration = 266 mg ÷ 4 ≈ 66.5 mg
Answer: 66.5 mg every 6 hours
Explanation: Multiply weight by dose, divide by doses.

Problem 176: A patient weighing 75 kg is prescribed 30 mg/kg/day divided into three doses. Calculate the dose per administration.
Solution:
Step 1: Total dose = 30 mg/kg × 75 kg = 2250 mg
Step 2: Dose per administration = 2250 mg ÷ 3 = 750 mg
Answer: 750 mg every 8 hours
Explanation: Multiply weight by dose, divide by doses.

Problem 177: A medication dose of 0.8 mg/kg/day is ordered for a 16 kg child. Calculate the total daily dose.
Solution:
Step 1: Total dose = 0.8 mg/kg × 16 kg = 12.8 mg

Answer: 12.8 mg per day
Explanation: Multiply weight by dose.

Problem 178: Calculate the dose per administration for a 65 kg patient prescribed 4 mg/kg/day divided into two doses.
Solution:
Step 1: Total dose = 4 mg/kg × 65 kg = 260 mg
Step 2: Dose per administration = 260 mg ÷ 2 = 130 mg
Answer: 130 mg every 12 hours
Explanation: Multiply weight by dose, divide by doses.

Problem 179: A child weighing 9 kg is prescribed 12 mg/kg/day divided into three doses. What is the dose per administration?
Solution:
Step 1: Total dose = 12 mg/kg × 9 kg = 108 mg
Step 2: Dose per administration = 108 mg ÷ 3 = 36 mg
Answer: 36 mg every 8 hours
Explanation: Multiply weight by dose, divide by doses.

Problem 180: Calculate the total daily dose for a 32 kg patient prescribed 5 mg/kg/day.
Solution:
Step 1: Total dose = 5 mg/kg × 32 kg = 160 mg
Answer: 160 mg per day
Explanation: Multiply weight by dose.

Problem 181: A medication is ordered at 2.2 mg/kg/day for a 27 kg child, divided into four doses. Calculate dose per administration.
Solution:
Step 1: Total dose = 2.2 mg/kg × 27 kg = 59.4 mg

Step 2: Dose per administration = 59.4 mg ÷ 4 = 14.85 mg
Answer: 14.85 mg every 6 hours
Explanation: Multiply weight by dose, divide by doses.

Problem 182: A 55 kg patient needs 15 mg/kg/day divided into three doses. What is the dose per administration?
Solution:
Step 1: Total dose = 15 mg/kg × 55 kg = 825 mg
Step 2: Dose per administration = 825 mg ÷ 3 = 275 mg
Answer: 275 mg every 8 hours
Explanation: Multiply weight by dose, divide by doses.

Problem 183: A medication is prescribed at 6 mg/kg/day for a 70 kg patient in two doses. What is the dose per administration?
Solution:
Step 1: Total dose = 6 mg/kg × 70 kg = 420 mg
Step 2: Dose per administration = 420 mg ÷ 2 = 210 mg
Answer: 210 mg every 12 hours
Explanation: Multiply weight by dose, divide by doses.

Problem 184: A child weighing 11 kg is ordered 10 mg/kg/day divided into four doses. What is the dose per administration?
Solution:
Step 1: Total dose = 10 mg/kg × 11 kg = 110 mg
Step 2: Dose per administration = 110 mg ÷ 4 = 27.5 mg
Answer: 27.5 mg every 6 hours
Explanation: Multiply weight by dose, divide by doses.

Problem 185: Calculate total daily dose for a 45 kg patient prescribed 25 mg/kg/day.

Solution:
Step 1: Total dose = 25 mg/kg × 45 kg = 1125 mg
Answer: 1125 mg per day
Explanation: Multiply weight by dose.

Problem 186: A medication dose of 0.5 mg/kg/day is ordered for a patient weighing 18 kg. Calculate total dose.
Solution:
Step 1: Total dose = 0.5 mg/kg × 18 kg = 9 mg
Answer: 9 mg per day
Explanation: Multiply weight by dose.

Problem 187: Calculate dose per administration for a 70 kg patient prescribed 60 mg/kg/day divided into three doses.
Solution:
Step 1: Total dose = 60 mg/kg × 70 kg = 4200 mg
Step 2: Dose per administration = 4200 mg ÷ 3 = 1400 mg
Answer: 1400 mg every 8 hours
Explanation: Multiply weight by dose, divide by doses.

Problem 188: A patient weighing 55 kg is prescribed 8 mg/kg/day divided into two doses. Calculate dose per administration.
Solution:
Step 1: Total dose = 8 mg/kg × 55 kg = 440 mg
Step 2: Dose per administration = 440 mg ÷ 2 = 220 mg
Answer: 220 mg every 12 hours
Explanation: Multiply weight by dose, divide by doses.

Problem 189: A child weighing 22 kg is ordered 20 mg/kg/day divided into four doses. Calculate dose per administration.

Solution:
Step 1: Total dose = 20 mg/kg × 22 kg = 440 mg
Step 2: Dose per administration = 440 mg ÷ 4 = 110 mg
Answer: 110 mg every 6 hours
Explanation: Multiply weight by dose, divide by doses.

Problem 190: A patient weighs 10 kg and is prescribed 2.5 mg/kg/day. Calculate total daily dose.
Solution:
Step 1: Total dose = 2.5 mg/kg × 10 kg = 25 mg
Answer: 25 mg per day
Explanation: Multiply weight by dose.

Problem 191: A medication is ordered at 3 mg/kg/day for a 40 kg patient in two doses. Calculate dose per administration.
Solution:
Step 1: Total dose = 3 mg/kg × 40 kg = 120 mg
Step 2: Dose per administration = 120 mg ÷ 2 = 60 mg
Answer: 60 mg every 12 hours
Explanation: Multiply weight by dose, divide by doses.

Problem 192: Calculate dose per administration for a 50 kg patient prescribed 1.2 mg/kg/day divided into three doses.
Solution:
Step 1: Total dose = 1.2 mg/kg × 50 kg = 60 mg
Step 2: Dose per administration = 60 mg ÷ 3 = 20 mg
Answer: 20 mg every 8 hours
Explanation: Multiply weight by dose, divide by doses.

Problem 193: A child weighs 12 kg and is ordered 10 mg/kg/day divided into two doses. Calculate dose per administration.
Solution:
Step 1: Total dose = 10 mg/kg × 12 kg = 120 mg
Step 2: Dose per administration = 120 mg ÷ 2 = 60 mg
Answer: 60 mg every 12 hours
Explanation: Multiply weight by dose, divide by doses.

Problem 194: A medication is prescribed at 7 mg/kg/day for a 38 kg

patient divided into four doses. Calculate dose per administration.
Solution:
Step 1: Total dose = 7 mg/kg × 38 kg = 266 mg
Step 2: Dose per administration = 266 mg ÷ 4 = 66.5 mg
Answer: 66.5 mg every 6 hours
Explanation: Multiply weight by dose, divide by doses.

Problem 195: A 75 kg patient is prescribed 30 mg/kg/day divided into three doses. Calculate dose per administration.
Solution:
Step 1: Total dose = 30 mg/kg × 75 kg = 2250 mg
Step 2: Dose per administration = 2250 mg ÷ 3 = 750 mg
Answer: 750 mg every 8 hours
Explanation: Multiply weight by dose, divide by doses.

Problem 196: A dose of 0.8 mg/kg/day is ordered for a 16 kg child. Calculate total daily dose.
Solution:
Step 1: Total dose = 0.8 mg/kg × 16 kg = 12.8 mg
Answer: 12.8 mg per day
Explanation: Multiply weight by dose.

Problem 197: Calculate dose per administration for a 65 kg patient prescribed 4 mg/kg/day divided into two doses.
Solution:
Step 1: Total dose = 4 mg/kg × 65 kg = 260 mg
Step 2: Dose per administration = 260 mg ÷ 2 = 130 mg
Answer: 130 mg every 12 hours
Explanation: Multiply weight by dose, divide by doses.

Problem 198: A child weighing 9 kg is prescribed 12 mg/kg/day divided into three doses. Calculate dose per administration.
Solution:
Step 1: Total dose = 12 mg/kg × 9 kg = 108 mg
Step 2: Dose per administration = 108 mg ÷ 3 = 36 mg
Answer: 36 mg every 8 hours
Explanation: Multiply weight by dose, divide by doses.

Problem 199: Calculate total daily dose for a 32 kg patient prescribed 5 mg/kg/day.
Solution:
Step 1: Total dose = 5 mg/kg × 32 kg = 160 mg
Answer: 160 mg per day
Explanation: Multiply weight by dose.

Problem 200: A medication is ordered at 2.2 mg/kg/day for a 27 kg child divided into four doses. Calculate dose per administration.
Solution:
Step 1: Total dose = 2.2 mg/kg × 27 kg = 59.4 mg
Step 2: Dose per administration = 59.4 mg ÷ 4 = 14.85 mg
Answer: 14.85 mg every 6 hours
Explanation: Multiply weight by dose, divide by doses.

Category 5: IV Flow Rates (gtt/min)

Problem 201: You must infuse 1000 mL of fluid over 8 hours using a 15 gtt/mL set. What is the flow rate in drops per minute?
Solution:
Step 1: Convert hours to minutes: 8 × 60 = 480 minutes
Step 2: Calculate mL per minute: 1000 ÷ 480 = 2.08 mL/min
Step 3: Calculate drops per minute: 2.08 × 15 = 31.25 ≈ 31 gtt/min
Answer: 31 drops per minute
Explanation: Calculate mL/min, then multiply by drop factor.

Problem 202: Infuse 500 mL over 4 hours with a 20 gtt/mL set. Calculate the drops per minute.
Solution:
Step 1: Convert hours to minutes: 4 × 60 = 240 minutes
Step 2: Calculate mL per minute: 500 ÷ 240 = 2.08 mL/min
Step 3: Calculate drops per minute: 2.08 × 20 = 41.67 ≈ 42 gtt/min
Answer: 42 drops per minute
Explanation: Multiply mL/min by drop factor.

Problem 203: You have 750 mL to infuse over 6 hours using a 10 gtt/mL set. What is the flow rate in gtt/min?
Solution:
Step 1: 6 hours = 360 minutes
Step 2: mL per minute: 750 ÷ 360 = 2.08 mL/min
Step 3: Drops per minute: 2.08 × 10 = 20.8 ≈ 21 gtt/min
Answer: 21 drops per minute
Explanation: Convert time, calculate mL/min and multiply by drop factor.

Problem 204: Infuse 1200 mL over 10 hours with a 60 gtt/mL set. Find drops per minute.
Solution:
Step 1: 10 hours = 600 minutes
Step 2: mL per minute: 1200 ÷ 600 = 2 mL/min
Step 3: Drops per minute: 2 × 60 = 120 gtt/min
Answer: 120 drops per minute
Explanation: Calculate mL/min then multiply by drop factor.

Problem 205: Infuse 250 mL over 30 minutes using a 15 gtt/mL set. Calculate flow rate in drops per minute.
Solution:
Step 1: 30 minutes total
Step 2: mL per minute: 250 ÷ 30 = 8.33 mL/min
Step 3: Drops per minute: 8.33 × 15 = 125 gtt/min
Answer: 125 drops per minute
Explanation: Divide volume by minutes, multiply by drop factor.

Problem 206: You need to infuse 500 mL in 3 hours using a 20 gtt/mL set. What is the drops per minute?
Solution:
Step 1: 3 hours = 180 minutes
Step 2: mL per minute: 500 ÷ 180 ≈ 2.78 mL/min
Step 3: Drops per minute: 2.78 × 20 ≈ 56 gtt/min
Answer: 56 drops per minute
Explanation: Calculate mL/min and multiply by drop factor.

Problem 207: Infuse 600 mL over 5 hours using a 10 gtt/mL set. Calculate drops per minute.
Solution:
Step 1: 5 hours = 300 minutes
Step 2: mL per minute: 600 ÷ 300 = 2 mL/min

163

Step 3: Drops per minute: $2 \times 10 = 20$ gtt/min
Answer: 20 drops per minute
Explanation: Multiply mL/min by drop factor.

Problem 208: Infuse 900 mL over 9 hours with a 15 gtt/mL set. Find drops per minute.
Solution:
Step 1: 9 hours = 540 minutes
Step 2: mL per minute: $900 \div 540 \approx 1.67$ mL/min
Step 3: Drops per minute: $1.67 \times 15 = 25$ gtt/min
Answer: 25 drops per minute
Explanation: Convert volume to mL/min, multiply by drop factor.

Problem 209: A patient requires 1000 mL over 24 hours via 60 gtt/mL set. Calculate the drops per minute.
Solution:
Step 1: 24 hours = 1440 minutes
Step 2: mL per minute: $1000 \div 1440 \approx 0.694$ mL/min
Step 3: Drops per minute: $0.694 \times 60 \approx 41.6 \approx 42$ gtt/min
Answer: 42 drops per minute
Explanation: Calculate mL/min and multiply by drop factor.

Problem 210: Infuse 100 mL over 15 minutes with a 20 gtt/mL set. Calculate drops per minute.
Solution:
Step 1: 15 minutes total
Step 2: mL per minute: $100 \div 15 = 6.67$ mL/min
Step 3: Drops per minute: $6.67 \times 20 = 133.4 \approx 133$ gtt/min
Answer: 133 drops per minute
Explanation: Calculate volume per minute, multiply by drop factor.

Problem 211: Infuse 1500 mL over 12 hours using a 60 gtt/mL set. Calculate drops per minute.
Solution:
Step 1: Convert hours to minutes: $12 \times 60 = 720$ minutes
Step 2: Calculate mL per minute: $1500 \div 720 \approx 2.08$ mL/min
Step 3: Calculate drops per minute: $2.08 \times 60 = 125$ gtt/min
Answer: 125 drops per minute
Explanation: Calculate mL/min and multiply by drop factor.

Problem 212: You need to infuse 400 mL over 3 hours using a 15 gtt/mL set. What is the drops per minute?
Solution:
Step 1: 3 hours = 180 minutes
Step 2: mL per minute: $400 \div 180 \approx 2.22$ mL/min
Step 3: Drops per minute: $2.22 \times 15 \approx 33$ gtt/min
Answer: 33 drops per minute
Explanation: Calculate volume per minute then multiply by drop factor.

Problem 213: Infuse 1000 mL over 16 hours with a 20 gtt/mL set. Find drops per minute.
Solution:
Step 1: 16 hours = 960 minutes
Step 2: mL per minute: $1000 \div 960 \approx 1.04$ mL/min
Step 3: Drops per minute: $1.04 \times 20 \approx 21$ gtt/min
Answer: 21 drops per minute
Explanation: Calculate mL/min and multiply by drop factor.

Problem 214: Infuse 800 mL over 4 hours using a 10 gtt/mL set. Calculate drops per minute.
Solution:
Step 1: 4 hours = 240 minutes

Step 2: mL per minute: 800 ÷ 240 ≈ 3.33 mL/min
Step 3: Drops per minute: 3.33 × 10 = 33 gtt/min
Answer: 33 drops per minute
Explanation: Calculate mL/min and multiply by drop factor.

Problem 215: Infuse 2000 mL over 24 hours using a 60 gtt/mL set. Calculate drops per minute.
Solution:
Step 1: 24 hours = 1440 minutes
Step 2: mL per minute: 2000 ÷ 1440 ≈ 1.39 mL/min
Step 3: Drops per minute: 1.39 × 60 ≈ 83 gtt/min
Answer: 83 drops per minute
Explanation: Calculate mL/min and multiply by drop factor.

Problem 216: You must infuse 300 mL over 1.5 hours with a 15 gtt/mL set. Find drops per minute.
Solution:
Step 1: 1.5 hours = 90 minutes
Step 2: mL per minute: 300 ÷ 90 = 3.33 mL/min
Step 3: Drops per minute: 3.33 × 15 = 50 gtt/min
Answer: 50 drops per minute
Explanation: Calculate mL/min and multiply by drop factor.

Problem 217: Infuse 1250 mL over 10 hours with a 20 gtt/mL set. Calculate drops per minute.
Solution:
Step 1: 10 hours = 600 minutes
Step 2: mL per minute: 1250 ÷ 600 ≈ 2.08 mL/min
Step 3: Drops per minute: 2.08 × 20 = 42 gtt/min
Answer: 42 drops per minute
Explanation: Calculate mL/min and multiply by drop factor.

Problem 218: Infuse 600 mL over 5 hours using a 15 gtt/mL set. Calculate drops per minute.
Solution:
Step 1: 5 hours = 300 minutes
Step 2: mL per minute: 600 ÷ 300 = 2 mL/min
Step 3: Drops per minute: 2 × 15 = 30 gtt/min
Answer: 30 drops per minute
Explanation: Calculate mL/min and multiply by drop factor.

Problem 219: A fluid volume of 750 mL is to be infused over 6 hours using a 60 gtt/mL set. Calculate drops per minute.
Solution:
Step 1: 6 hours = 360 minutes
Step 2: mL per minute: 750 ÷ 360 ≈ 2.08 mL/min
Step 3: Drops per minute: 2.08 × 60 = 125 gtt/min
Answer: 125 drops per minute
Explanation: Calculate mL/min and multiply by drop factor.

Problem 220: You need to infuse 400 mL over 2 hours using a 10 gtt/mL set. Calculate drops per minute.
Solution:
Step 1: 2 hours = 120 minutes
Step 2: mL per minute: 400 ÷ 120 = 3.33 mL/min
Step 3: Drops per minute: 3.33 × 10 = 33 gtt/min
Answer: 33 drops per minute
Explanation: Calculate mL/min and multiply by drop factor.

Problem 221: Infuse 900 mL over 3 hours with a 15 gtt/mL set. Calculate drops per minute.
Solution:

Step 1: 3 hours = 180 minutes
Step 2: mL per minute: 900 ÷ 180 = 5 mL/min
Step 3: Drops per minute: 5 × 15 = 75 gtt/min
Answer: 75 drops per minute
Explanation: Calculate mL/min and multiply by drop factor.

Problem 222: A patient requires 1000 mL over 20 hours with a 60 gtt/mL set. Calculate drops per minute.
Solution:
Step 1: 20 hours = 1200 minutes
Step 2: mL per minute: 1000 ÷ 1200 = 0.833 mL/min
Step 3: Drops per minute: 0.833 × 60 = 50 gtt/min
Answer: 50 drops per minute
Explanation: Calculate mL/min and multiply by drop factor.

Problem 223: Infuse 500 mL over 1 hour using a 15 gtt/mL set. Calculate drops per minute.
Solution:
Step 1: 1 hour = 60 minutes
Step 2: mL per minute: 500 ÷ 60 ≈ 8.33 mL/min
Step 3: Drops per minute: 8.33 × 15 ≈ 125 gtt/min
Answer: 125 drops per minute
Explanation: Calculate mL/min and multiply by drop factor.

Problem 224: Infuse 350 mL over 30 minutes with a 20 gtt/mL set. Calculate drops per minute.
Solution:
Step 1: 30 minutes total
Step 2: mL per minute: 350 ÷ 30 ≈ 11.67 mL/min
Step 3: Drops per minute: 11.67 × 20 = 233 gtt/min
Answer: 233 drops per minute
Explanation: Calculate mL/min and multiply by drop factor.

Problem 225: You must infuse 150 mL over 45 minutes using a 60 gtt/mL set. Calculate drops per minute.
Solution:
Step 1: 45 minutes total
Step 2: mL per minute: 150 ÷ 45 = 3.33 mL/min
Step 3: Drops per minute: 3.33 × 60 = 200 gtt/min
Answer: 200 drops per minute
Explanation: Calculate mL/min and multiply by drop factor.

Problem 226: Infuse 800 mL over 10 hours with a 10 gtt/mL set. Calculate drops per minute.
Solution:
Step 1: 10 hours = 600 minutes
Step 2: mL per minute: 800 ÷ 600 = 1.33 mL/min
Step 3: Drops per minute: 1.33 × 10 = 13 gtt/min
Answer: 13 drops per minute
Explanation: Calculate mL/min and multiply by drop factor.

Problem 227: A fluid is to be infused: 600 mL over 8 hours using a 20 gtt/mL set. Calculate drops per minute.
Solution:
Step 1: 8 hours = 480 minutes
Step 2: mL per minute: 600 ÷ 480 = 1.25 mL/min
Step 3: Drops per minute: 1.25 × 20 = 25 gtt/min
Answer: 25 drops per minute
Explanation: Calculate mL/min and multiply by drop factor.

Problem 228: You must infuse 900 mL over 9 hours using a 15 gtt/mL set. Calculate drops per minute.
Solution:

Step 1: 9 hours = 540 minutes
Step 2: mL per minute: 900 ÷ 540 = 1.67 mL/min
Step 3: Drops per minute: 1.67 × 15 = 25 gtt/min
Answer: 25 drops per minute
Explanation: Calculate mL/min and multiply by drop factor.

Problem 229: Infuse 1000 mL over 15 hours with a 60 gtt/mL set. Calculate drops per minute.
Solution:
Step 1: 15 hours = 900 minutes
Step 2: mL per minute: 1000 ÷ 900 = 1.11 mL/min
Step 3: Drops per minute: 1.11 × 60 = 67 gtt/min
Answer: 67 drops per minute
Explanation: Calculate mL/min and multiply by drop factor.

Problem 230: You have 300 mL to infuse over 2 hours with a 20 gtt/mL set. Calculate drops per minute.
Solution:
Step 1: 2 hours = 120 minutes
Step 2: mL per minute: 300 ÷ 120 = 2.5 mL/min
Step 3: Drops per minute: 2.5 × 20 = 50 gtt/min
Answer: 50 drops per minute
Explanation: Calculate mL/min and multiply by drop factor.

Problem 231: Infuse 450 mL over 6 hours with a 15 gtt/mL set. Calculate drops per minute.
Solution:
Step 1: 6 hours = 360 minutes
Step 2: mL per minute: 450 ÷ 360 = 1.25 mL/min
Step 3: Drops per minute: 1.25 × 15 = 19 gtt/min
Answer: 19 drops per minute
Explanation: Calculate mL/min and multiply by drop factor.

Problem 232: Infuse 100 mL over 10 minutes using a 60 gtt/mL set. Calculate drops per minute.
Solution:
Step 1: 10 minutes total
Step 2: mL per minute: 100 ÷ 10 = 10 mL/min
Step 3: Drops per minute: 10 × 60 = 600 gtt/min
Answer: 600 drops per minute
Explanation: Calculate mL/min and multiply by drop factor.

Problem 233: A patient needs 550 mL infused over 5 hours using a 10 gtt/mL set. Calculate drops per minute.
Solution:
Step 1: 5 hours = 300 minutes
Step 2: mL per minute: 550 ÷ 300 ≈ 1.83 mL/min
Step 3: Drops per minute: 1.83 × 10 = 18 gtt/min
Answer: 18 drops per minute
Explanation: Calculate mL/min and multiply by drop factor.

Problem 234: Infuse 1000 mL over 7 hours using a 20 gtt/mL set. Calculate drops per minute.
Solution:
Step 1: 7 hours = 420 minutes
Step 2: mL per minute: 1000 ÷ 420 ≈ 2.38 mL/min
Step 3: Drops per minute: 2.38 × 20 = 48 gtt/min
Answer: 48 drops per minute
Explanation: Calculate mL/min and multiply by drop factor.

Problem 235: You must infuse 1250 mL over 10 hours with a 15 gtt/mL set. Calculate drops per minute.
Solution:

171

Step 1: 10 hours = 600 minutes
Step 2: mL per minute: 1250 ÷ 600 ≈ 2.08 mL/min
Step 3: Drops per minute: 2.08 × 15 = 31 gtt/min
Answer: 31 drops per minute
Explanation: Calculate mL/min and multiply by drop factor.

Problem 236: Infuse 700 mL over 3.5 hours with a 60 gtt/mL set. Calculate drops per minute.
Solution:
Step 1: 3.5 hours = 210 minutes
Step 2: mL per minute: 700 ÷ 210 ≈ 3.33 mL/min
Step 3: Drops per minute: 3.33 × 60 = 200 gtt/min
Answer: 200 drops per minute
Explanation: Calculate mL/min and multiply by drop factor.

Problem 237: Infuse 400 mL over 50 minutes with a 20 gtt/mL set. Calculate drops per minute.
Solution:
Step 1: 50 minutes total
Step 2: mL per minute: 400 ÷ 50 = 8 mL/min
Step 3: Drops per minute: 8 × 20 = 160 gtt/min
Answer: 160 drops per minute
Explanation: Calculate mL/min and multiply by drop factor.

Problem 238: You have 1000 mL to infuse over 18 hours with a 15 gtt/mL set. Calculate drops per minute.
Solution:
Step 1: 18 hours = 1080 minutes
Step 2: mL per minute: 1000 ÷ 1080 ≈ 0.93 mL/min
Step 3: Drops per minute: 0.93 × 15 ≈ 14 gtt/min
Answer: 14 drops per minute
Explanation: Calculate mL/min and multiply by drop factor.

Problem 239: Infuse 600 mL over 2 hours with a 10 gtt/mL set. Calculate drops per minute.
Solution:
Step 1: 2 hours = 120 minutes
Step 2: mL per minute: 600 ÷ 120 = 5 mL/min
Step 3: Drops per minute: 5 × 10 = 50 gtt/min
Answer: 50 drops per minute
Explanation: Calculate mL/min and multiply by drop factor.

Problem 240: A patient needs 900 mL infused over 4.5 hours using a 20 gtt/mL set. Calculate drops per minute.
Solution:
Step 1: 4.5 hours = 270 minutes
Step 2: mL per minute: 900 ÷ 270 ≈ 3.33 mL/min
Step 3: Drops per minute: 3.33 × 20 = 67 gtt/min
Answer: 67 drops per minute
Explanation: Calculate mL/min and multiply by drop factor.

Problem 241: Infuse 750 mL over 9 hours with a 15 gtt/mL set. Calculate drops per minute.
Solution:
Step 1: 9 hours = 540 minutes
Step 2: mL per minute: 750 ÷ 540 ≈ 1.39 mL/min
Step 3: Drops per minute: 1.39 × 15 ≈ 21 gtt/min
Answer: 21 drops per minute
Explanation: Calculate mL/min and multiply by drop factor.

Problem 242: Infuse 100 mL over 25 minutes with a 60 gtt/mL set. Calculate drops per minute.
Solution:

Step 1: 25 minutes total
Step 2: mL per minute: 100 ÷ 25 = 4 mL/min
Step 3: Drops per minute: 4 × 60 = 240 gtt/min
Answer: 240 drops per minute
Explanation: Calculate mL/min and multiply by drop factor.

Problem 243: You have 1200 mL to infuse over 14 hours using a 10 gtt/mL set. Calculate drops per minute.
Solution:
Step 1: 14 hours = 840 minutes
Step 2: mL per minute: 1200 ÷ 840 ≈ 1.43 mL/min
Step 3: Drops per minute: 1.43 × 10 = 14 gtt/min
Answer: 14 drops per minute
Explanation: Calculate mL/min and multiply by drop factor.

Problem 244: Infuse 2000 mL over 16 hours with a 20 gtt/mL set. Calculate drops per minute.
Solution:
Step 1: 16 hours = 960 minutes
Step 2: mL per minute: 2000 ÷ 960 ≈ 2.08 mL/min
Step 3: Drops per minute: 2.08 × 20 = 42 gtt/min
Answer: 42 drops per minute
Explanation: Calculate mL/min and multiply by drop factor.

Problem 245: Infuse 300 mL over 1 hour with a 15 gtt/mL set. Calculate drops per

minute.
Solution:
Step 1: 1 hour = 60 minutes
Step 2: mL per minute: 300 ÷ 60 = 5 mL/min
Step 3: Drops per minute: 5 × 15 = 75 gtt/min

Answer: 75 drops per minute
Explanation: Calculate mL/min and multiply by drop factor.

Problem 246: Infuse 450 mL over 2 hours with a 60 gtt/mL set. Calculate drops per minute.
Solution:
Step 1: 2 hours = 120 minutes
Step 2: mL per minute: 450 ÷ 120 = 3.75 mL/min
Step 3: Drops per minute: 3.75 × 60 = 225 gtt/min
Answer: 225 drops per minute
Explanation: Calculate mL/min and multiply by drop factor.

Problem 247: A patient requires 800 mL infused over 6 hours with a 10 gtt/mL set. Calculate drops per minute.
Solution:
Step 1: 6 hours = 360 minutes
Step 2: mL per minute: 800 ÷ 360 ≈ 2.22 mL/min
Step 3: Drops per minute: 2.22 × 10 = 22 gtt/min
Answer: 22 drops per minute
Explanation: Calculate mL/min and multiply by drop factor.

Problem 248: Infuse 500 mL over 4 hours with a 20 gtt/mL set. Calculate drops per minute.
Solution:
Step 1: 4 hours = 240 minutes
Step 2: mL per minute: 500 ÷ 240 ≈ 2.08 mL/min
Step 3: Drops per minute: 2.08 × 20 = 42 gtt/min
Answer: 42 drops per minute
Explanation: Calculate mL/min and multiply by drop factor.

Problem 249: You have 700 mL to infuse over 5 hours using a 15 gtt/mL set. Calculate drops per minute.
Solution:
Step 1: 5 hours = 300 minutes
Step 2: mL per minute: 700 ÷ 300 ≈ 2.33 mL/min
Step 3: Drops per minute: 2.33 × 15 = 35 gtt/min
Answer: 35 drops per minute
Explanation: Calculate mL/min and multiply by drop factor.

Problem 250: Infuse 1000 mL over 7 hours using a 60 gtt/mL set. Calculate drops per minute.
Solution:
Step 1: 7 hours = 420 minutes
Step 2: mL per minute: 1000 ÷ 420 ≈ 2.38 mL/min
Step 3: Drops per minute: 2.38 × 60 = 143 gtt/min
Answer: 143 drops per minute
Explanation: Calculate mL/min and multiply by drop factor.

Category 6: IV Pump Rates (mL/hr)

Problem 251: Infuse 1000 mL over 10 hours. What is the pump rate in mL/hr?
Solution:
Step 1: Rate = Total volume ÷ Time = 1000 mL ÷ 10 hr = 100 mL/hr
Answer: 100 mL/hr
Explanation: Divide total volume by infusion time.

Problem 252: A patient needs 500 mL infused over 2.5 hours. What is the pump rate?
Solution:
Step 1: Rate = 500 mL ÷ 2.5 hr = 200 mL/hr
Answer: 200 mL/hr
Explanation: Divide volume by time.

Problem 253: Infuse 750 mL over 5 hours. Calculate mL/hr rate.
Solution:
Step 1: Rate = 750 mL ÷ 5 hr = 150 mL/hr
Answer: 150 mL/hr
Explanation: Divide volume by infusion time.

Problem 254: A patient requires 300 mL infused in 45 minutes. What is the pump rate in mL/hr?
Solution:
Step 1: Convert time to hours: 45 min = 0.75 hr
Step 2: Rate = 300 mL ÷ 0.75 hr = 400 mL/hr
Answer: 400 mL/hr
Explanation: Convert minutes to hours, then divide volume by time.

Problem 255: Infuse 1200 mL over 8 hours. Find the pump rate.
Solution:
Step 1: Rate = 1200 mL ÷ 8 hr = 150 mL/hr
Answer: 150 mL/hr
Explanation: Divide total volume by time.

Problem 256: You need to infuse 200 mL over 30 minutes. Calculate the pump rate in mL/hr.
Solution:
Step 1: Convert time: 30 min = 0.5 hr
Step 2: Rate = 200 mL ÷ 0.5 hr = 400 mL/hr
Answer: 400 mL/hr
Explanation: Convert minutes to hours, then divide volume by time.

Problem 257: Infuse 1000 mL over 20 hours. What is the pump rate?
Solution:
Step 1: Rate = 1000 mL ÷ 20 hr = 50 mL/hr
Answer: 50 mL/hr
Explanation: Divide volume by infusion time.

Problem 258: A patient is ordered 250 mL to be infused in 1 hour and 15 minutes. What is the pump rate in mL/hr?
Solution:
Step 1: Convert time to hours: 1 hr 15 min = 1.25 hr
Step 2: Rate = 250 mL ÷ 1.25 hr = 200 mL/hr
Answer: 200 mL/hr
Explanation: Convert time and divide volume by time.

Problem 259: Infuse 900 mL over 9 hours. Calculate pump rate.
Solution:
Step 1: Rate = 900 mL ÷ 9 hr = 100 mL/hr
Answer: 100 mL/hr
Explanation: Divide volume by time.

Problem 260: You need to deliver 1500 mL in 12 hours. What should the pump rate be?
Solution:
Step 1: Rate = 1500 mL ÷ 12 hr = 125 mL/hr
Answer: 125 mL/hr
Explanation: Divide total volume by hours.

Problem 261: Infuse 350 mL over 45 minutes. Calculate pump rate in mL/hr.
Solution:
Step 1: Convert time: 45 min = 0.75 hr
Step 2: Rate = 350 mL ÷ 0.75 hr = 466.67 mL/hr
Answer: 467 mL/hr (rounded)
Explanation: Convert time and divide volume by time.

Problem 262: A medication is ordered to infuse 600 mL over 6 hours. Find the pump rate.
Solution:
Step 1: Rate = 600 mL ÷ 6 hr = 100 mL/hr
Answer: 100 mL/hr
Explanation: Divide volume by time.

Problem 263: Infuse 800 mL over 10 hours. Calculate mL/hr rate.
Solution:

Step 1: Rate = 800 mL ÷ 10 hr = 80 mL/hr
Answer: 80 mL/hr
Explanation: Divide total volume by hours.

Problem 264: You have 400 mL to infuse over 2 hours and 30 minutes. What is the pump rate?
Solution:
Step 1: Convert time: 2 hr 30 min = 2.5 hr
Step 2: Rate = 400 mL ÷ 2.5 hr = 160 mL/hr
Answer: 160 mL/hr
Explanation: Convert time and divide volume.

Problem 265: Infuse 100 mL over 20 minutes. Calculate the pump rate in mL/hr.
Solution:
Step 1: Convert time: 20 min = 0.333 hr
Step 2: Rate = 100 mL ÷ 0.333 hr ≈ 300 mL/hr
Answer: 300 mL/hr
Explanation: Convert minutes to hours and divide volume.

Problem 266: Infuse 1200 mL over 15 hours. Calculate the rate.
Solution:
Step 1: Rate = 1200 mL ÷ 15 hr = 80 mL/hr
Answer: 80 mL/hr
Explanation: Divide volume by time.

Problem 267: A patient needs 700 mL infused in 3.5 hours. What is the pump rate?
Solution:
Step 1: Rate = 700 mL ÷ 3.5 hr = 200 mL/hr

Answer: 200 mL/hr
Explanation: Divide volume by hours.

Problem 268: You are to infuse 500 mL over 45 minutes. Calculate mL/hr rate.
Solution:
Step 1: Convert time: 45 min = 0.75 hr
Step 2: Rate = 500 mL ÷ 0.75 hr = 666.67 mL/hr
Answer: 667 mL/hr (rounded)
Explanation: Convert time and divide volume.

Problem 269: Infuse 1500 mL over 24 hours. Calculate the pump rate.
Solution:
Step 1: Rate = 1500 mL ÷ 24 hr = 62.5 mL/hr
Answer: 62.5 mL/hr
Explanation: Divide volume by hours.

Problem 270: A medication is ordered to be infused 600 mL over 5 hours. Calculate the pump rate.
Solution:
Step 1: Rate = 600 mL ÷ 5 hr = 120 mL/hr
Answer: 120 mL/hr
Explanation: Divide volume by time.

Problem 271: You have to infuse 450 mL over 3 hours. Calculate mL/hr rate.
Solution:
Step 1: Rate = 450 mL ÷ 3 hr = 150 mL/hr

Answer: 150 mL/hr
Explanation: Divide volume by hours.

Problem 272: Infuse 1000 mL over 18 hours. Find the pump rate.
Solution:
Step 1: Rate = 1000 mL ÷ 18 hr ≈ 55.56 mL/hr
Answer: 55.56 mL/hr
Explanation: Divide volume by time.

Problem 273: You need to infuse 350 mL over 90 minutes. Calculate mL/hr rate.
Solution:
Step 1: Convert time: 90 min = 1.5 hr
Step 2: Rate = 350 mL ÷ 1.5 hr ≈ 233.33 mL/hr
Answer: 233.33 mL/hr
Explanation: Convert time and divide volume.

Problem 274: Infuse 800 mL over 7 hours. Calculate pump rate.
Solution:
Step 1: Rate = 800 mL ÷ 7 hr ≈ 114.29 mL/hr
Answer: 114.29 mL/hr
Explanation: Divide volume by hours.

Problem 275: You have 1000 mL to infuse over 4 hours and 30 minutes. What is the pump rate?
Solution:
Step 1: Convert time: 4 hr 30 min = 4.5 hr
Step 2: Rate = 1000 mL ÷ 4.5 hr ≈ 222.22 mL/hr
Answer: 222.22 mL/hr
Explanation: Convert time and divide volume.

Category 7: Reconstitution of Powdered Drugs

Problem 276: A vial contains 500 mg of powdered drug. You add 5 mL of diluent. What is the concentration in mg/mL?
Solution:
Step 1: Total drug = 500 mg
Step 2: Total volume after reconstitution = 5 mL
Step 3: Concentration = 500 mg ÷ 5 mL = 100 mg/mL
Answer: 100 mg/mL
Explanation: Divide total drug by total volume to find concentration.

Problem 277: A vial contains 1 g (1000 mg) of powder. After adding 10 mL diluent, what is the concentration in mg/mL?
Solution:
Step 1: Total drug = 1000 mg
Step 2: Total volume = 10 mL
Step 3: Concentration = 1000 mg ÷ 10 mL = 100 mg/mL
Answer: 100 mg/mL
Explanation: Divide drug amount by volume.

Problem 278: After reconstituting a 250 mg powder with 5 mL diluent, what is the concentration?
Solution:
Step 1: Total drug = 250 mg
Step 2: Total volume = 5 mL
Step 3: Concentration = 250 mg ÷ 5 mL = 50 mg/mL
Answer: 50 mg/mL
Explanation: Divide drug amount by volume.

Problem 279: You need 200 mg of medication. The vial concentration after reconstitution is 100 mg/mL. How many milliliters should you draw?
Solution:
Step 1: Volume = Dose ÷ Concentration = 200 mg ÷ 100 mg/mL = 2 mL
Answer: 2 mL
Explanation: Divide desired dose by concentration.

Problem 280: A vial contains 1.5 g powder. Reconstitute with 15 mL of diluent. What is the concentration in mg/mL?
Solution:
Step 1: Convert 1.5 g to mg = 1.5 × 1000 = 1500 mg
Step 2: Total volume = 15 mL
Step 3: Concentration = 1500 mg ÷ 15 mL = 100 mg/mL
Answer: 100 mg/mL
Explanation: Divide drug amount by total volume.

Problem 281: You reconstitute 500 mg powder with 10 mL diluent. How many milliliters contain 300 mg?
Solution:
Step 1: Concentration = 500 mg ÷ 10 mL = 50 mg/mL
Step 2: Volume for 300 mg = 300 mg ÷ 50 mg/mL = 6 mL
Answer: 6 mL
Explanation: Calculate concentration, then use to find required volume.

Problem 282: After reconstitution, the concentration is 25 mg/mL. How many milliliters deliver 125 mg?
Solution:
Step 1: Volume = Dose ÷ Concentration = 125 mg ÷ 25 mg/mL = 5 mL

Answer: 5 mL
Explanation: Divide dose by concentration.

Problem 283: A 2 g vial is reconstituted with 20 mL. What is the concentration in mg/mL?
Solution:
Step 1: Convert 2 g to mg = 2000 mg
Step 2: Concentration = 2000 mg ÷ 20 mL = 100 mg/mL
Answer: 100 mg/mL
Explanation: Divide drug amount by volume.

Problem 284: You need to administer 150 mg. The vial concentration after reconstitution is 75 mg/mL. How many milliliters do you draw?
Solution:
Step 1: Volume = Dose ÷ Concentration = 150 mg ÷ 75 mg/mL = 2 mL
Answer: 2 mL
Explanation: Divide dose by concentration.

Problem 285: A vial with 1 g powder is reconstituted with 8 mL diluent. What is the concentration?
Solution:
Step 1: Convert 1 g to mg = 1000 mg
Step 2: Concentration = 1000 mg ÷ 8 mL = 125 mg/mL
Answer: 125 mg/mL
Explanation: Divide drug amount by volume.

Problem 286: After reconstitution, concentration is 40 mg/mL. How many milliliters contain 80 mg?
Solution:

Step 1: Volume = Dose ÷ Concentration = 80 mg ÷ 40 mg/mL = 2 mL
Answer: 2 mL
Explanation: Divide dose by concentration.

Problem 287: A 500 mg vial is reconstituted with 4 mL diluent. What is the concentration?
Solution:
Step 1: Concentration = 500 mg ÷ 4 mL = 125 mg/mL
Answer: 125 mg/mL
Explanation: Divide drug amount by volume.

Problem 288: You must administer 250 mg from a vial concentration of 125 mg/mL. How many milliliters do you draw?
Solution:
Step 1: Volume = Dose ÷ Concentration = 250 mg ÷ 125 mg/mL = 2 mL
Answer: 2 mL
Explanation: Divide dose by concentration.

Problem 289: A vial contains 750 mg powder reconstituted with 15 mL diluent. What is the concentration?
Solution:
Step 1: Concentration = 750 mg ÷ 15 mL = 50 mg/mL
Answer: 50 mg/mL
Explanation: Divide drug amount by volume.

Problem 290: You need 300 mg from a vial concentration of 50 mg/mL. How many milliliters should you administer?
Solution:
Step 1: Volume = Dose ÷ Concentration = 300 mg ÷ 50 mg/mL = 6

mL
Answer: 6 mL
Explanation: Divide dose by concentration.

Problem 291: A 2.5 g vial is reconstituted with 20 mL. What is the concentration?
Solution:
Step 1: Convert 2.5 g to mg = 2500 mg
Step 2: Concentration = 2500 mg ÷ 20 mL = 125 mg/mL
Answer: 125 mg/mL
Explanation: Divide drug amount by volume.

Problem 292: After reconstitution, concentration is 30 mg/mL. How many milliliters deliver 90 mg?
Solution:
Step 1: Volume = Dose ÷ Concentration = 90 mg ÷ 30 mg/mL = 3 mL
Answer: 3 mL
Explanation: Divide dose by concentration.

Problem 293: A vial with 600 mg powder is reconstituted with 12 mL diluent. What is the concentration?
Solution:
Step 1: Concentration = 600 mg ÷ 12 mL = 50 mg/mL
Answer: 50 mg/mL
Explanation: Divide drug amount by volume.

Problem 294: You must give 150 mg from a vial with concentration 50 mg/mL. How many milliliters do you administer?
Solution:
Step 1: Volume = Dose ÷ Concentration = 150 mg ÷ 50 mg/mL = 3

187

mL
Answer: 3 mL
Explanation: Divide dose by concentration.

Problem 295: A vial contains 800 mg of powder reconstituted with 8 mL diluent. What is the concentration?
Solution:
Step 1: Concentration = 800 mg ÷ 8 mL = 100 mg/mL
Answer: 100 mg/mL
Explanation: Divide drug amount by volume.

Problem 296: You need 200 mg from a vial concentration of 100 mg/mL. How many milliliters do you draw?
Solution:
Step 1: Volume = Dose ÷ Concentration = 200 mg ÷ 100 mg/mL = 2 mL
Answer: 2 mL
Explanation: Divide dose by concentration.

Problem 297: A 1.2 g vial is reconstituted with 12 mL. What is the concentration?
Solution:
Step 1: Convert 1.2 g to mg = 1200 mg
Step 2: Concentration = 1200 mg ÷ 12 mL = 100 mg/mL
Answer: 100 mg/mL
Explanation: Divide drug amount by volume.

Problem 298: After reconstitution, concentration is 60 mg/mL. How many milliliters provide 180 mg?
Solution:

Step 1: Volume = Dose ÷ Concentration = 180 mg ÷ 60 mg/mL = 3 mL
Answer: 3 mL
Explanation: Divide dose by concentration.

Problem 299: A vial with 900 mg powder is reconstituted with 9 mL. What is the concentration?
Solution:
Step 1: Concentration = 900 mg ÷ 9 mL = 100 mg/mL
Answer: 100 mg/mL
Explanation: Divide drug amount by volume.

Problem 300: You must administer 250 mg from a vial with concentration 125 mg/mL. How many milliliters are needed?
Solution:
Step 1: Volume = Dose ÷ Concentration = 250 mg ÷ 125 mg/mL = 2 mL
Answer: 2 mL
Explanation: Divide dose by concentration.

Category 8: Time and Rate Adjustments Calculations

Problem 301: A patient requires an infusion of 1000 mL over 10 hours. After 5 hours, the rate is doubled. How many milliliters will be infused in total after 10 hours?

Solution:

Step 1: Calculate rate for first 5 hours: 1000 mL ÷ 10 hr = 100 mL/hr

Step 2: Volume infused in first 5 hours: 100 mL/hr × 5 hr = 500 mL

Step 3: New rate after doubling: 100 × 2 = 200 mL/hr

Step 4: Volume infused in last 5 hours: 200 mL/hr × 5 hr = 1000 mL

Step 5: Total volume infused: 500 + 1000 = 1500 mL

Answer: 1500 mL

Explanation: Calculate volumes infused at different rates, sum for total.

Problem 302: A medication order requires 400 mg/day given as 100 mg every 6 hours. How many doses will the patient receive in 24 hours?

Solution:

Step 1: Number of doses = 24 hr ÷ 6 hr = 4 doses

Answer: 4 doses

Explanation: Divide total hours by dosing interval.

Problem 303: A loading dose of 500 mg is given over 30 minutes, followed by a maintenance dose of 250 mg every 8 hours. How much medication is administered in 24 hours?

Solution:

Step 1: Number of maintenance doses: 24 hr ÷ 8 hr = 3 doses

Step 2: Total maintenance dose: 250 mg × 3 = 750 mg

Step 3: Total medication in 24 hr: 500 mg + 750 mg = 1250 mg

Answer: 1250 mg

Explanation: Add loading dose to cumulative maintenance doses.

Problem 304: An infusion is started at 50 mL/hr. After 4 hours, the rate is increased by 20 mL/hr. How much fluid is infused in 8 hours?

Solution:

Step 1: Volume infused first 4 hours: 50 mL/hr × 4 hr = 200 mL

Step 2: New rate: 50 + 20 = 70 mL/hr

Step 3: Volume infused last 4 hours: 70 mL/hr × 4 hr = 280 mL

Step 4: Total volume: 200 + 280 = 480 mL

Answer: 480 mL

Explanation: Calculate volumes at different rates, add.

Problem 305: A drug is dosed at 2 mg/kg/day in divided doses every 8 hours for a 25 kg patient. How much drug is given per dose?

Solution:

Step 1: Total daily dose: 2 mg/kg × 25 kg = 50 mg

Step 2: Number of doses: 24 ÷ 8 = 3 doses

Step 3: Dose per administration: 50 mg ÷ 3 ≈ 16.67 mg

Answer: 16.67 mg per dose

Explanation: Calculate total daily dose and divide by doses per day.

Problem 306: A medication is titrated by increasing the dose by 5 mg every 12 hours, starting at 10 mg. What will the dose be after 36 hours?

Solution:

Step 1: Number of 12-hr increments in 36 hr: 36 ÷ 12 = 3

Step 2: Total increase: 5 mg × 3 = 15 mg

Step 3: Dose after 36 hours: 10 mg + 15 mg = 25 mg

Answer: 25 mg

Explanation: Calculate increments, add to initial dose.

Problem 307: An IV infusion of 800 mL is running at 100 mL/hr. How long will it take to finish?
Solution:
Step 1: Time = Volume ÷ Rate = 800 mL ÷ 100 mL/hr = 8 hours
Answer: 8 hours
Explanation: Divide total volume by infusion rate.

Problem 308: A medication requires a maintenance dose of 300 mg/day. If divided into 3 doses, what is the dose per administration?
Solution:
Step 1: Dose per administration: 300 mg ÷ 3 = 100 mg
Answer: 100 mg per dose
Explanation: Divide daily dose by number of doses.

Problem 309: A continuous infusion is running at 60 mL/hr. After 6 hours, the rate is decreased by 15 mL/hr. How much fluid is infused in 12 hours?
Solution:
Step 1: Volume first 6 hours: 60 mL/hr × 6 hr = 360 mL
Step 2: New rate: 60 - 15 = 45 mL/hr
Step 3: Volume next 6 hours: 45 mL/hr × 6 hr = 270 mL
Step 4: Total volume: 360 + 270 = 630 mL
Answer: 630 mL
Explanation: Calculate volumes at different rates, sum.

Problem 310: A medication has a half-life of 8 hours. If a patient receives 100 mg at 8 AM, how much remains at 4 PM?
Solution:
Step 1: Time elapsed: 8 hours (8 AM to 4 PM)
Step 2: Remaining dose = 100 mg × ½ = 50 mg

192

Answer: 50 mg
Explanation: Half of the drug remains after one half-life.

Problem 311: A drug is administered every 6 hours. If the first dose is given at 6 AM, when is the fourth dose given?
Solution:
Step 1: Doses at 6 AM, 12 PM, 6 PM, and 12 AM
Answer: 12 AM (midnight)
Explanation: Add multiples of dosing interval to initial dose time.

Problem 312: A medication order requires tapering the dose by 10 mg every 2 days, starting at 80 mg. What is the dose on day 7?
Solution:
Step 1: Number of 2-day intervals in 7 days = $7 \div 2 = 3$ intervals (ignore remainder)
Step 2: Total decrease: $10 \text{ mg} \times 3 = 30 \text{ mg}$
Step 3: Dose on day 7: 80 mg - 30 mg = 50 mg
Answer: 50 mg
Explanation: Calculate total decrease over intervals.

Problem 313: A patient is prescribed a medication at 5 mg/kg/day divided every 6 hours. Patient weighs 40 kg. What is the dose per administration?
Solution:
Step 1: Total daily dose = $5 \text{ mg/kg} \times 40 \text{ kg} = 200 \text{ mg}$
Step 2: Number of doses per day: $24 \div 6 = 4$
Step 3: Dose per administration: $200 \text{ mg} \div 4 = 50 \text{ mg}$
Answer: 50 mg per dose
Explanation: Calculate total daily dose and divide by doses.

Problem 314: A medication is infused at 150 mL/hr for 3 hours, then increased to 200 mL/hr for 5 hours. How much total fluid is infused?
Solution:
Step 1: Volume at 150 mL/hr: 150 × 3 = 450 mL
Step 2: Volume at 200 mL/hr: 200 × 5 = 1000 mL
Step 3: Total volume: 450 + 1000 = 1450 mL
Answer: 1450 mL
Explanation: Calculate volume for each rate, then sum.

Problem 315: A patient is ordered 100 mg every 8 hours. How many doses will they receive in 48 hours?
Solution:
Step 1: Number of doses = 48 ÷ 8 = 6 doses
Answer: 6 doses
Explanation: Divide total hours by dosing interval.

Problem 316: A patient is receiving 200 mL/hr infusion. After 3 hours, the rate decreases by 50 mL/hr. How much fluid is infused in 7 hours?
Solution:
Step 1: Volume in first 3 hours: 200 × 3 = 600 mL
Step 2: New rate: 200 - 50 = 150 mL/hr
Step 3: Volume in remaining 4 hours: 150 × 4 = 600 mL
Step 4: Total volume: 600 + 600 = 1200 mL
Answer: 1200 mL
Explanation: Calculate volume at each rate, then sum.

Problem 317: A medication requires 300 mg/day in 3 equal doses. How many milligrams per dose?
Solution:
Step 1: 300 mg ÷ 3 = 100 mg

Answer: 100 mg per dose
Explanation: Divide daily dose by number of doses.

Problem 318: You administer a loading dose of 800 mg, followed by maintenance doses of 200 mg every 8 hours. How much drug is given in 24 hours?
Solution:
Step 1: Number of maintenance doses: $24 \div 8 = 3$
Step 2: Total maintenance dose: $200 \times 3 = 600$ mg
Step 3: Total in 24 hours: $800 + 600 = 1400$ mg
Answer: 1400 mg
Explanation: Add loading dose to total maintenance doses.

Problem 319: An IV infusion runs at 50 mL/hr for 6 hours, then at 70 mL/hr for 4 hours. What is total volume infused?
Solution:
Step 1: Volume at 50 mL/hr: $50 \times 6 = 300$ mL
Step 2: Volume at 70 mL/hr: $70 \times 4 = 280$ mL
Step 3: Total volume: $300 + 280 = 580$ mL
Answer: 580 mL
Explanation: Calculate volume per rate, sum totals.

Problem 320: A medication with half-life of 6 hours is given at 200 mg at 8 AM. How much remains at 2 PM?
Solution:
Step 1: Time elapsed: 6 hours
Step 2: Remaining amount $= 200$ mg $\times \frac{1}{2} = 100$ mg
Answer: 100 mg
Explanation: One half-life reduces drug by half.

Problem 321: A patient needs 250 mg every 12 hours. How many doses in 48 hours?
Solution:
Step 1: Number of doses = 48 ÷ 12 = 4 doses
Answer: 4 doses
Explanation: Divide total time by dosing interval.

Problem 322: A drug is titrated upward by 10 mg every 24 hours starting at 50 mg. What is the dose on day 4?
Solution:
Step 1: Number of increases by day 4 = 3 (days 2,3,4)
Step 2: Total increase = 10 × 3 = 30 mg
Step 3: Dose on day 4 = 50 + 30 = 80 mg
Answer: 80 mg
Explanation: Add increments to starting dose.

Problem 323: An infusion runs 80 mL/hr for 5 hours then is reduced to 60 mL/hr for 7 hours. Total volume infused?
Solution:
Step 1: Volume first 5 hr: 80 × 5 = 400 mL
Step 2: Volume next 7 hr: 60 × 7 = 420 mL
Step 3: Total volume: 400 + 420 = 820 mL
Answer: 820 mL
Explanation: Calculate volume at each rate and sum.

Problem 324: A patient weighing 60 kg is prescribed 10 mg/kg/day divided into 4 doses. Dose per administration?
Solution:
Step 1: Total daily dose = 10 × 60 = 600 mg
Step 2: Dose per administration = 600 ÷ 4 = 150 mg
Answer: 150 mg
Explanation: Calculate total dose and divide.

Problem 325: A loading dose of 400 mg is given followed by 100 mg every 6 hours. How much drug in 24 hours?
Solution:
Step 1: Number of maintenance doses: $24 \div 6 = 4$
Step 2: Maintenance dose total $= 100 \times 4 = 400$ mg
Step 3: Total dose $= 400 + 400 = 800$ mg
Answer: 800 mg
Explanation: Add loading dose to maintenance doses.

Problem 326: A medication is given as 300 mg/day in divided doses every 8 hours. Dose per administration?
Solution:
Step 1: Number of doses $= 24 \div 8 = 3$
Step 2: Dose $= 300 \div 3 = 100$ mg
Answer: 100 mg
Explanation: Divide total dose by number of doses.

Problem 327: An IV infusion of 1200 mL runs at 100 mL/hr for 6 hours, then increased to 150 mL/hr for 4 hours. Total infused?
Solution:
Step 1: Volume first 6 hr: $100 \times 6 = 600$ mL
Step 2: Volume next 4 hr: $150 \times 4 = 600$ mL
Step 3: Total volume: $600 + 600 = 1200$ mL
Answer: 1200 mL
Explanation: Calculate volume infused in each period.

Problem 328: A medication dose is 50 mg every 12 hours. How many doses in 36 hours?
Solution:
Step 1: Number of doses $= 36 \div 12 = 3$

Answer: 3 doses
Explanation: Divide total time by dosing interval.

Problem 329: An infusion rate is decreased by 25 mL/hr every 4 hours, starting at 150 mL/hr. What is the rate at 12 hours?
Solution:
Step 1: Number of decreases: $12 \div 4 = 3$
Step 2: Total decrease: $25 \times 3 = 75$ mL/hr
Step 3: New rate: 150 - 75 = 75 mL/hr
Answer: 75 mL/hr
Explanation: Calculate total decrease and subtract.

Problem 330: A drug with half-life 4 hours has a 300 mg dose at 6 AM. How much remains at 2 PM?
Solution:
Step 1: Time elapsed: 8 hours = 2 half-lives
Step 2: Remaining = $300 \times (\frac{1}{2})^2 = 300 \times \frac{1}{4} = 75$ mg
Answer: 75 mg
Explanation: Two half-lives reduce dose by 75%.

Problem 331: A medication is dosed at 4 mg/kg/day for a 70 kg patient, divided every 6 hours. Dose per administration?
Solution:
Step 1: Total daily dose = $4 \times 70 = 280$ mg
Step 2: Doses per day = $24 \div 6 = 4$
Step 3: Dose per administration = $280 \div 4 = 70$ mg
Answer: 70 mg
Explanation: Calculate total and divide by doses.

Problem 332: An IV drip runs at 60 mL/hr for 5 hours, then at 40 mL/hr for 3 hours. How much fluid is infused?
Solution:
Step 1: Volume first 5 hr: 60 × 5 = 300 mL
Step 2: Volume next 3 hr: 40 × 3 = 120 mL
Step 3: Total volume: 300 + 120 = 420 mL
Answer: 420 mL
Explanation: Add volumes infused at each rate.

Problem 333: A patient receives 600 mg/day divided into 3 doses every 8 hours. What is each dose?
Solution:
Step 1: Dose per administration = 600 ÷ 3 = 200 mg
Answer: 200 mg
Explanation: Divide total dose by number of doses.

Problem 334: After 2 doses of 400 mg, a drug is tapered by 50 mg every 12 hours. What is the dose after 3 days?
Solution:
Step 1: Number of 12-hr periods in 3 days = 3 × 24 ÷ 12 = 6
Step 2: Total taper: 50 × 6 = 300 mg
Step 3: Dose after taper = 400 - 300 = 100 mg
Answer: 100 mg
Explanation: Subtract cumulative taper amount.

Problem 335: A loading dose of 500 mg is followed by 150 mg every 6 hours. How much drug is given in 24 hours?
Solution:
Step 1: Number of doses: 24 ÷ 6 = 4
Step 2: Total maintenance: 150 × 4 = 600 mg
Step 3: Total dose: 500 + 600 = 1100 mg

Answer: 1100 mg
Explanation: Sum loading and maintenance doses.

Problem 336: A patient weighing 55 kg is prescribed 3 mg/kg/day divided into 3 doses. Dose per administration?
Solution:
Step 1: Total dose = 3 × 55 = 165 mg
Step 2: Dose per administration = 165 ÷ 3 = 55 mg
Answer: 55 mg
Explanation: Calculate total and divide.

Problem 337: An infusion runs at 75 mL/hr for 7 hours, then is stopped. Total volume infused?
Solution:
Step 1: Volume = 75 × 7 = 525 mL
Answer: 525 mL
Explanation: Multiply rate by time.

Problem 338: A drug with half-life 12 hours is dosed 100 mg at 8 AM. How much remains at 8 PM?
Solution:
Step 1: Time elapsed: 12 hr = 1 half-life
Step 2: Remaining = 100 × ½ = 50 mg
Answer: 50 mg
Explanation: One half-life halves the dose.

Problem 339: A patient is ordered 200 mg every 4 hours. How many doses in 24 hours?
Solution:
Step 1: Number of doses = 24 ÷ 4 = 6

Answer: 6 doses
Explanation: Divide total time by dosing interval.

Problem 340: A medication is increased by 5 mg every day starting at 10 mg. What is the dose on day 6?
Solution:
Step 1: Number of increases by day 6 = 5
Step 2: Total increase = 5 × 5 = 25 mg
Step 3: Dose on day 6 = 10 + 25 = 35 mg
Answer: 35 mg
Explanation: Add daily increases to initial dose.

Problem 341: Infuse 1800 mL over 24 hours. What is the pump rate?
Solution:
Step 1: Rate = 1800 ÷ 24 = 75 mL/hr
Answer: 75 mL/hr
Explanation: Divide volume by time.

Problem 342: You have to infuse 900 mL over 6 hours. Calculate mL/hr.
Solution:
Step 1: Rate = 900 ÷ 6 = 150 mL/hr
Answer: 150 mL/hr
Explanation: Divide volume by time.

Problem 343: A patient receives 150 mg every 12 hours. How many doses in 48 hours?
Solution:
Step 1: Number of doses = 48 ÷ 12 = 4

Answer: 4 doses
Explanation: Divide total time by dosing interval.

Problem 344: A medication is tapered by 10 mg every 24 hours, starting at 80 mg. What is the dose after 5 days?
Solution:
Step 1: Total taper: $10 \times 5 = 50$ mg
Step 2: Dose after taper = 80 - 50 = 30 mg
Answer: 30 mg
Explanation: Subtract cumulative taper.

Problem 345: A medication is dosed at 2 mg/kg/day for a 40 kg patient, divided every 8 hours. Dose per administration?
Solution:
Step 1: Total dose = $2 \times 40 = 80$ mg
Step 2: Number doses = $24 \div 8 = 3$
Step 3: Dose per administration = $80 \div 3 \approx 26.67$ mg
Answer: 26.67 mg
Explanation: Calculate total dose and divide.

Problem 346: An infusion runs at 100 mL/hr for 8 hours, then at 120 mL/hr for 4 hours. Total volume?
Solution:
Step 1: Volume first 8 hr: $100 \times 8 = 800$ mL
Step 2: Volume next 4 hr: $120 \times 4 = 480$ mL
Step 3: Total volume: 800 + 480 = 1280 mL
Answer: 1280 mL
Explanation: Calculate each segment and add.

Problem 347: A patient needs 450 mg/day in 3 doses every 8 hours. Dose per administration?
Solution:
Step 1: Dose per administration = 450 ÷ 3 = 150 mg
Answer: 150 mg
Explanation: Divide daily dose by doses per day.

Problem 348: You increase a drug dose by 25% daily starting from 100 mg. What is the dose on day 3?
Solution:
Step 1: Day 1: 100 mg
Step 2: Day 2: 100 + 25% of 100 = 125 mg
Step 3: Day 3: 125 + 25% of 125 = 125 + 31.25 = 156.25 mg
Answer: 156.25 mg
Explanation: Increase dose by 25% each day.

Problem 349: A medication is infused at 200 mL/hr for 2 hours, then 150 mL/hr for 3 hours. Total volume infused?
Solution:
Step 1: Volume first 2 hr: 200 × 2 = 400 mL
Step 2: Volume next 3 hr: 150 × 3 = 450 mL
Step 3: Total volume: 400 + 450 = 850 mL
Answer: 850 mL
Explanation: Calculate volumes and add.

Problem 350: A patient is prescribed 100 mg every 4 hours. How many doses in 72 hours?
Solution:
Step 1: Number of doses = 72 ÷ 4 = 18
Answer: 18 doses
Explanation: Divide total hours by dosing interval.

Certainly! I will create **three separate subcategories** under **Special Population Dosage Calculations**, each with **50 questions**, totaling **150 questions** from 351 to 500:

Category 9: Pediatrics Dosage Calculations

Problem 351: A 4-year-old child weighs 16 kg. The dose is 10 mg/kg/day divided into 4 doses. What is the dose per administration?
Solution:
Step 1: Total daily dose = 10 × 16 = 160 mg
Step 2: Dose per administration = 160 ÷ 4 = 40 mg
Answer: 40 mg per dose
Explanation: Multiply weight by dose per kg and divide by number of doses.

Problem 352: A medication dose is 5 mg/kg/day for a 10 kg infant. Calculate total daily dose.
Solution:
Step 1: Total dose = 5 × 10 = 50 mg
Answer: 50 mg per day
Explanation: Multiply weight by mg/kg dose.

Problem 353: A pediatric patient weighs 22 kg and requires 7 mg/kg/day in 3 doses. What is each dose?
Solution:
Step 1: Total dose = 7 × 22 = 154 mg
Step 2: Dose per administration = 154 ÷ 3 ≈ 51.33 mg
Answer: 51.33 mg per dose
Explanation: Calculate total and divide.

Problem 354: A newborn weighing 3.5 kg needs 15 mg/kg/day. Calculate the total daily dose.
Solution:
Step 1: Total dose = 15 × 3.5 = 52.5 mg

Answer: 52.5 mg
Explanation: Multiply weight by dose per kg.

Problem 355: A 6-year-old weighing 18 kg needs 12 mg/kg/day divided into 2 doses. What is dose per administration?
Solution:
Step 1: Total dose = 12 × 18 = 216 mg
Step 2: Dose per dose = 216 ÷ 2 = 108 mg
Answer: 108 mg per dose
Explanation: Multiply weight by dose, divide by number of doses.

Problem 356: A child is prescribed 500 mg/day in 5 divided doses. How much per dose?
Solution:
Step 1: Dose per administration = 500 ÷ 5 = 100 mg
Answer: 100 mg per dose
Explanation: Divide total daily dose by number of doses.

Problem 357: A medication order is 6 mg/kg/day for a 14 kg child in 3 doses. Dose per administration?
Solution:
Step 1: Total dose = 6 × 14 = 84 mg
Step 2: Dose per dose = 84 ÷ 3 = 28 mg
Answer: 28 mg per dose
Explanation: Multiply and divide accordingly.

Problem 358: Calculate total dose for a 9 kg infant prescribed 20 mg/kg/day.
Solution:
Step 1: Total dose = 20 × 9 = 180 mg

Answer: 180 mg per day
Explanation: Multiply weight by dose.

Problem 359: A 12-year-old weighing 40 kg needs 10 mg/kg/day divided into 4 doses. Dose per administration?
Solution:
Step 1: Total dose = 10 × 40 = 400 mg
Step 2: Dose per administration = 400 ÷ 4 = 100 mg
Answer: 100 mg per dose
Explanation: Multiply and divide.

Problem 360: A 3-year-old (14 kg) requires 5 mg/kg/day in 2 doses. Calculate dose per dose.
Solution:
Step 1: Total dose = 5 × 14 = 70 mg
Step 2: Dose per administration = 70 ÷ 2 = 35 mg
Answer: 35 mg per dose
Explanation: Multiply and divide.

Problem 361: A child weighs 25 kg and is prescribed 8 mg/kg/day divided into 4 doses. What is the dose per administration?
Solution:
Step 1: Total dose = 8 × 25 = 200 mg
Step 2: Dose per administration = 200 ÷ 4 = 50 mg
Answer: 50 mg per dose
Explanation: Multiply weight by dose then divide by number of doses.

Problem 362: A 5-year-old child weighing 18 kg requires 15 mg/kg/day. What is the total daily dose?

Solution:
Step 1: Total dose = 15 × 18 = 270 mg
Answer: 270 mg per day
Explanation: Multiply weight by dose per kg.

Problem 363: A pediatric dose is 7 mg/kg/day divided into 3 doses for a 10 kg infant. Dose per administration?
Solution:
Step 1: Total dose = 7 × 10 = 70 mg
Step 2: Dose per dose = 70 ÷ 3 ≈ 23.33 mg
Answer: 23.33 mg per dose
Explanation: Calculate total then divide.

Problem 364: An infant weighing 5 kg is prescribed 20 mg/kg/day. Calculate total daily dose.
Solution:
Step 1: Total dose = 20 × 5 = 100 mg
Answer: 100 mg
Explanation: Multiply weight by mg/kg.

Problem 365: A child weighing 30 kg needs 9 mg/kg/day divided into 3 doses. Dose per administration?
Solution:
Step 1: Total dose = 9 × 30 = 270 mg
Step 2: Dose per dose = 270 ÷ 3 = 90 mg
Answer: 90 mg per dose
Explanation: Multiply and divide.

Problem 366: A child is prescribed 450 mg/day divided into 5 doses. What is the dose per administration?

Solution:
Step 1: Dose per dose = 450 ÷ 5 = 90 mg
Answer: 90 mg per dose
Explanation: Divide total dose by doses.

Problem 367: A 2-year-old child weighing 12 kg needs 12 mg/kg/day. What is the total daily dose?
Solution:
Step 1: Total dose = 12 × 12 = 144 mg
Answer: 144 mg
Explanation: Multiply weight by dose.

Problem 368: A pediatric patient requires 6 mg/kg/day divided into 3 doses. Patient weighs 14 kg. Calculate dose per administration.
Solution:
Step 1: Total dose = 6 × 14 = 84 mg
Step 2: Dose per dose = 84 ÷ 3 = 28 mg
Answer: 28 mg per dose
Explanation: Multiply and divide.

Problem 369: Calculate total daily dose for a 16 kg child prescribed 10 mg/kg/day.
Solution:
Step 1: Total dose = 10 × 16 = 160 mg
Answer: 160 mg
Explanation: Multiply weight by dose.

Problem 370: A child weighs 20 kg and is prescribed 14 mg/kg/day divided into 4 doses. Calculate dose per administration.
Solution:

Step 1: Total dose = 14 × 20 = 280 mg
Step 2: Dose per dose = 280 ÷ 4 = 70 mg
Answer: 70 mg per dose
Explanation: Multiply and divide.

Problem 371: A pediatric dose is 5 mg/kg/day for a 22 kg child divided into 2 doses. What is the dose per administration?
Solution:
Step 1: Total dose = 5 × 22 = 110 mg
Step 2: Dose per dose = 110 ÷ 2 = 55 mg
Answer: 55 mg per dose
Explanation: Multiply and divide.

Problem 372: A 3-year-old weighing 13 kg needs 18 mg/kg/day. Calculate the total daily dose.
Solution:
Step 1: Total dose = 18 × 13 = 234 mg
Answer: 234 mg
Explanation: Multiply weight by dose.

Problem 373: A medication is ordered as 7 mg/kg/day in 3 doses for a child weighing 25 kg. Dose per administration?
Solution:
Step 1: Total dose = 7 × 25 = 175 mg
Step 2: Dose per dose = 175 ÷ 3 ≈ 58.33 mg
Answer: 58.33 mg per dose
Explanation: Multiply and divide.

Problem 374: A 6-year-old child (22 kg) is prescribed 10 mg/kg/day divided into 4 doses. Calculate dose per administration.

Solution:
Step 1: Total dose = 10 × 22 = 220 mg
Step 2: Dose per dose = 220 ÷ 4 = 55 mg
Answer: 55 mg per dose
Explanation: Multiply and divide.

Problem 375: Calculate total daily dose for a 9 kg infant prescribed 15 mg/kg/day.
Solution:
Step 1: Total dose = 15 × 9 = 135 mg
Answer: 135 mg
Explanation: Multiply weight by dose.

Problem 376: A child weighing 18 kg is prescribed 8 mg/kg/day divided into 3 doses. Dose per administration?
Solution:
Step 1: Total dose = 8 × 18 = 144 mg
Step 2: Dose per dose = 144 ÷ 3 = 48 mg
Answer: 48 mg per dose
Explanation: Multiply and divide.

Problem 377: A 5-year-old child weighing 20 kg needs 9 mg/kg/day divided into 2 doses. Calculate dose per administration.
Solution:
Step 1: Total dose = 9 × 20 = 180 mg
Step 2: Dose per dose = 180 ÷ 2 = 90 mg
Answer: 90 mg per dose
Explanation: Multiply and divide.

Problem 378: A medication is prescribed as 400 mg/day in 4 doses. Calculate dose per administration.
Solution:
Step 1: Dose per dose = 400 ÷ 4 = 100 mg
Answer: 100 mg per dose
Explanation: Divide total dose by doses.

Problem 379: A pediatric patient weighs 14 kg and is prescribed 12 mg/kg/day divided into 3 doses. Calculate dose per administration.
Solution:
Step 1: Total dose = 12 × 14 = 168 mg
Step 2: Dose per dose = 168 ÷ 3 = 56 mg
Answer: 56 mg per dose
Explanation: Multiply and divide.

Problem 380: A 10-year-old child weighing 30 kg needs 6 mg/kg/day divided into 4 doses. Dose per administration?
Solution:
Step 1: Total dose = 6 × 30 = 180 mg
Step 2: Dose per dose = 180 ÷ 4 = 45 mg
Answer: 45 mg per dose
Explanation: Multiply and divide.

Problem 381: A child weighs 7 kg and is prescribed 20 mg/kg/day divided into 3 doses. Calculate dose per administration.
Solution:
Step 1: Total dose = 20 × 7 = 140 mg
Step 2: Dose per dose = 140 ÷ 3 ≈ 46.67 mg
Answer: 46.67 mg per dose
Explanation: Multiply and divide.

Problem 382: Calculate total daily dose for a 13 kg infant prescribed 10 mg/kg/day.
Solution:
Step 1: Total dose = 10 × 13 = 130 mg
Answer: 130 mg
Explanation: Multiply weight by dose.

Problem 383: A pediatric dose is 5 mg/kg/day for a child weighing 16 kg divided into 2 doses. Dose per administration?
Solution:
Step 1: Total dose = 5 × 16 = 80 mg
Step 2: Dose per dose = 80 ÷ 2 = 40 mg
Answer: 40 mg per dose
Explanation: Multiply and divide.

Problem 384: A 3-year-old child weighing 12 kg requires 15 mg/kg/day divided into 3 doses. Calculate dose per administration.
Solution:
Step 1: Total dose = 15 × 12 = 180 mg
Step 2: Dose per dose = 180 ÷ 3 = 60 mg
Answer: 60 mg per dose
Explanation: Multiply and divide.

Problem 385: A medication is ordered as 500 mg/day in 5 divided doses. What is the dose per administration?
Solution:
Step 1: Dose per dose = 500 ÷ 5 = 100 mg
Answer: 100 mg per dose
Explanation: Divide total dose.

Problem 386: A child weighs 24 kg and is prescribed 9 mg/kg/day divided into 3 doses. Calculate dose per administration.
Solution:
Step 1: Total dose = 9 × 24 = 216 mg
Step 2: Dose per dose = 216 ÷ 3 = 72 mg
Answer: 72 mg per dose
Explanation: Multiply and divide.

Problem 387: A 5-year-old child weighing 18 kg needs 10 mg/kg/day divided into 4 doses. Dose per administration?
Solution:
Step 1: Total dose = 10 × 18 = 180 mg
Step 2: Dose per dose = 180 ÷ 4 = 45 mg
Answer: 45 mg per dose
Explanation: Multiply and divide.

Problem 388: Calculate total daily dose for a 6 kg infant prescribed 12 mg/kg/day.
Solution:
Step 1: Total dose = 12 × 6 = 72 mg
Answer: 72 mg
Explanation: Multiply weight by dose.

Problem 389: A pediatric dose is 8 mg/kg/day for a 15 kg child divided into 3 doses. Dose per administration?
Solution:
Step 1: Total dose = 8 × 15 = 120 mg
Step 2: Dose per dose = 120 ÷ 3 = 40 mg
Answer: 40 mg per dose
Explanation: Multiply and divide.

Problem 390: A child weighing 20 kg needs 11 mg/kg/day divided into 4 doses. Calculate dose per administration.
Solution:
Step 1: Total dose = 11 × 20 = 220 mg
Step 2: Dose per dose = 220 ÷ 4 = 55 mg
Answer: 55 mg per dose
Explanation: Multiply and divide.

Problem 391: A 2-year-old weighing 10 kg requires 14 mg/kg/day divided into 3 doses. Dose per administration?
Solution:
Step 1: Total dose = 14 × 10 = 140 mg
Step 2: Dose per dose = 140 ÷ 3 ≈ 46.67 mg
Answer: 46.67 mg per dose
Explanation: Multiply and divide.

Problem 392: Calculate total daily dose for a 13 kg child prescribed 9 mg/kg/day.
Solution:
Step 1: Total dose = 9 × 13 = 117 mg
Answer: 117 mg
Explanation: Multiply weight by dose.

Problem 393: A medication is ordered as 600 mg/day divided into 4 doses. Calculate dose per administration.
Solution:
Step 1: Dose per dose = 600 ÷ 4 = 150 mg
Answer: 150 mg per dose
Explanation: Divide total dose.

Problem 394: A child weighs 17 kg and is prescribed 10 mg/kg/day divided into 3 doses. Calculate dose per administration.
Solution:
Step 1: Total dose = 10 × 17 = 170 mg
Step 2: Dose per dose = 170 ÷ 3 ≈ 56.67 mg
Answer: 56.67 mg per dose
Explanation: Multiply and divide.

Problem 395: A 4-year-old weighing 15 kg needs 13 mg/kg/day divided into 4 doses. Dose per administration?
Solution:
Step 1: Total dose = 13 × 15 = 195 mg
Step 2: Dose per dose = 195 ÷ 4 = 48.75 mg
Answer: 48.75 mg per dose
Explanation: Multiply and divide.

Problem 396: A medication is ordered as 300 mg/day divided into 3 doses. What is the dose per administration?
Solution:
Step 1: Dose per dose = 300 ÷ 3 = 100 mg
Answer: 100 mg per dose
Explanation: Divide total dose.

Problem 397: A child weighing 22 kg is prescribed 12 mg/kg/day divided into 2 doses. Calculate dose per administration.
Solution:
Step 1: Total dose = 12 × 22 = 264 mg
Step 2: Dose per dose = 264 ÷ 2 = 132 mg
Answer: 132 mg per dose
Explanation: Multiply and divide.

Problem 398: Calculate total daily dose for a 14 kg child prescribed 10 mg/kg/day.
Solution:
Step 1: Total dose = 10 × 14 = 140 mg
Answer: 140 mg
Explanation: Multiply weight by dose.

Problem 399: A 3-year-old weighing 13 kg needs 8 mg/kg/day divided into 3 doses. Dose per administration?
Solution:
Step 1: Total dose = 8 × 13 = 104 mg
Step 2: Dose per dose = 104 ÷ 3 ≈ 34.67 mg
Answer: 34.67 mg per dose
Explanation: Multiply and divide.

Problem 400: A pediatric dose is 15 mg/kg/day for a 10 kg infant divided into 2 doses. Dose per administration?
Solution:
Step 1: Total dose = 15 × 10 = 150 mg
Step 2: Dose per dose = 150 ÷ 2 = 75 mg
Answer: 75 mg per dose
Explanation: Multiply and divide.

Category 10. Geriatrics Dosage Calculations

Problem 401: An 80-year-old patient is prescribed 400 mg/day. Due to decreased metabolism, reduce dose by 30%. What is the adjusted dose?
Solution:
Step 1: Calculate 30% of 400 mg: $0.30 \times 400 = 120$ mg
Step 2: Adjusted dose = 400 - 120 = 280 mg
Answer: 280 mg/day
Explanation: Apply percentage reduction due to age.

Problem 402: A standard adult dose is 250 mg. For a frail elderly patient, the dose is decreased by 25%. Calculate new dose.
Solution:
Step 1: 25% of 250 = $0.25 \times 250 = 62.5$ mg
Step 2: New dose = 250 - 62.5 = 187.5 mg
Answer: 187.5 mg
Explanation: Reduce dose by 25% for frailty.

Problem 403: An elderly patient takes 500 mg daily. After developing renal impairment, dose is cut by 40%. What is new dose?
Solution:
Step 1: 40% of 500 = 200 mg
Step 2: New dose = 500 - 200 = 300 mg
Answer: 300 mg/day
Explanation: Reduce dose due to renal impairment.

Problem 404: A geriatric patient on polypharmacy requires dose reduction by 20% from 600 mg. Calculate new dose.
Solution:
Step 1: 20% of 600 = 120 mg
Step 2: New dose = 600 - 120 = 480 mg
Answer: 480 mg
Explanation: Reduce dose due to polypharmacy risk.

Problem 405: A 75-year-old patient's usual dose is 100 mg twice daily. If dose is reduced by 15%, what is the new dose per administration?
Solution:
Step 1: 15% of 100 = 15 mg
Step 2: New dose = 100 - 15 = 85 mg
Answer: 85 mg per dose
Explanation: Reduce each dose by 15%.

Problem 406: An elderly patient requires 300 mg daily. Due to hepatic impairment, dose is decreased by 35%. Calculate adjusted dose.
Solution:
Step 1: 35% of 300 = 105 mg
Step 2: Adjusted dose = 300 - 105 = 195 mg
Answer: 195 mg/day
Explanation: Adjust dose for liver impairment.

Problem 407: Standard dose is 50 mg/day. In elderly patients, dose is reduced by 20%. What is the adjusted dose?
Solution:
Step 1: 20% of 50 = 10 mg
Step 2: Adjusted dose = 50 - 10 = 40 mg

Answer: 40 mg/day
Explanation: Reduce dose by 20%.

Problem 408: A geriatric patient requires 600 mg daily. Dose is decreased by 10% for age-related changes. What is the new dose?
Solution:
Step 1: 10% of 600 = 60 mg
Step 2: New dose = 600 - 60 = 540 mg
Answer: 540 mg/day
Explanation: Adjust dose accordingly.

Problem 409: Patient takes 400 mg daily, dose reduced by 50% for hepatic impairment. Calculate adjusted dose.
Solution:
Step 1: 50% of 400 = 200 mg
Step 2: New dose = 400 - 200 = 200 mg
Answer: 200 mg/day
Explanation: Significant reduction for liver issues.

Problem 410: An 85-year-old requires 200 mg/day, dose reduced by 25%. What is the adjusted dose?
Solution:
Step 1: 25% of 200 = 50 mg
Step 2: New dose = 200 - 50 = 150 mg
Answer: 150 mg/day
Explanation: Dose adjustment for age.

Problem 411: A 70-year-old patient is prescribed 100 mg twice daily. If reduced by 20%, what is the dose per administration?
Solution:

Step 1: 20% of 100 = 20 mg
Step 2: New dose = 100 - 20 = 80 mg
Answer: 80 mg per dose
Explanation: Dose reduced by 20%.

Problem 412: Usual dose is 300 mg daily. Due to frailty, reduce by 35%. Calculate new dose.
Solution:
Step 1: 35% of 300 = 105 mg
Step 2: New dose = 300 - 105 = 195 mg
Answer: 195 mg/day
Explanation: Reduce for frailty.

Problem 413: Elderly patient requires 400 mg daily. Reduce dose by 30% due to renal impairment. Adjusted dose?
Solution:
Step 1: 30% of 400 = 120 mg
Step 2: New dose = 400 - 120 = 280 mg
Answer: 280 mg/day
Explanation: Adjust dose accordingly.

Problem 414: Dose is 150 mg daily, reduce by 15% for age-related decline. Calculate new dose.
Solution:
Step 1: 15% of 150 = 22.5 mg
Step 2: New dose = 150 - 22.5 = 127.5 mg
Answer: 127.5 mg/day
Explanation: Reduce by percentage.

Problem 415: A medication requires 500 mg daily. Due to polypharmacy risk, reduce by 25%. What is new dose?
Solution:
Step 1: 25% of 500 = 125 mg
Step 2: New dose = 500 - 125 = 375 mg
Answer: 375 mg/day
Explanation: Dose reduction for safety.

Problem 416: An elderly patient's 200 mg dose is reduced by 10% for hepatic impairment. Adjusted dose?
Solution:
Step 1: 10% of 200 = 20 mg
Step 2: New dose = 200 - 20 = 180 mg
Answer: 180 mg/day
Explanation: Adjust for liver function.

Problem 417: Usual dose is 350 mg daily, reduced by 40% for renal issues. What is adjusted dose?
Solution:
Step 1: 40% of 350 = 140 mg
Step 2: New dose = 350 - 140 = 210 mg
Answer: 210 mg/day
Explanation: Reduce dose for kidney function.

Problem 418: Dose is 100 mg daily. Reduce by 20% for advanced age. Adjusted dose?
Solution:
Step 1: 20% of 100 = 20 mg
Step 2: New dose = 80 mg
Answer: 80 mg/day
Explanation: Dose reduction.

Problem 419: Patient takes 600 mg daily. Reduce by 15% for hepatic impairment. New dose?
Solution:
Step 1: 15% of 600 = 90 mg
Step 2: New dose = 600 - 90 = 510 mg
Answer: 510 mg/day
Explanation: Adjust dose.

Problem 420: Elderly patient's 250 mg dose is reduced by 35%. What is new dose?
Solution:
Step 1: 35% of 250 = 87.5 mg
Step 2: New dose = 162.5 mg
Answer: 162.5 mg
Explanation: Dose reduction.

Problem 421: Usual dose is 450 mg/day. Reduce by 25% for polypharmacy. Adjusted dose?
Solution:
Step 1: 25% of 450 = 112.5 mg
Step 2: New dose = 337.5 mg
Answer: 337.5 mg
Explanation: Reduce for safety.

Problem 422: A patient takes 800 mg daily, reduce by 30% for renal impairment. What is new dose?
Solution:
Step 1: 30% of 800 = 240 mg
Step 2: New dose = 560 mg

Answer: 560 mg/day
Explanation: Adjust for kidney function.

Problem 423: Elderly patient requires 100 mg daily, reduce dose by 10%. New dose?
Solution:
Step 1: 10% of 100 = 10 mg
Step 2: New dose = 90 mg
Answer: 90 mg/day
Explanation: Dose reduction.

Problem 424: A 300 mg dose is decreased by 40% for hepatic impairment. What is the new dose?
Solution:
Step 1: 40% of 300 = 120 mg
Step 2: New dose = 180 mg
Answer: 180 mg/day
Explanation: Adjust dose accordingly.

Problem 425: Dose is 500 mg daily, reduce by 20% for advanced age. New dose?
Solution:
Step 1: 20% of 500 = 100 mg
Step 2: New dose = 400 mg
Answer: 400 mg/day
Explanation: Dose reduction.

Problem 426: Elderly patient requires 350 mg, reduce by 15% due to frailty. New dose?
Solution:

Step 1: 15% of 350 = 52.5 mg
Step 2: New dose = 297.5 mg
Answer: 297.5 mg
Explanation: Reduce dose accordingly.

Problem 427: Usual dose 400 mg reduced by 30% for renal impairment. Adjusted dose?
Solution:
Step 1: 30% of 400 = 120 mg
Step 2: New dose = 280 mg
Answer: 280 mg/day
Explanation: Adjust dose for kidneys.

Problem 428: A patient requires 150 mg daily, reduce by 10% for age. New dose?
Solution:
Step 1: 10% of 150 = 15 mg
Step 2: New dose = 135 mg
Answer: 135 mg/day
Explanation: Dose reduction.

Problem 429: Dose is 600 mg, decrease by 25% for hepatic function. What is adjusted dose?
Solution:
Step 1: 25% of 600 = 150 mg
Step 2: New dose = 450 mg
Answer: 450 mg/day
Explanation: Reduce dose.

Problem 430: A 700 mg dose is decreased by 35% for renal impairment. Adjusted dose?
Solution:
Step 1: 35% of 700 = 245 mg
Step 2: New dose = 455 mg
Answer: 455 mg/day
Explanation: Reduce dose for kidneys.

Problem 431: Dose of 250 mg reduced by 20% for age. New dose?
Solution:
Step 1: 20% of 250 = 50 mg
Step 2: New dose = 200 mg
Answer: 200 mg/day
Explanation: Dose reduction.

Problem 432: A 300 mg dose reduced by 15% for frailty. Adjusted dose?
Solution:
Step 1: 15% of 300 = 45 mg
Step 2: New dose = 255 mg
Answer: 255 mg/day
Explanation: Adjust dose accordingly.

Problem 433: Patient requires 450 mg daily, reduce dose by 30%. New dose?
Solution:
Step 1: 30% of 450 = 135 mg
Step 2: New dose = 315 mg
Answer: 315 mg/day
Explanation: Dose adjustment.

Problem 434: Dose of 350 mg reduced by 10% for hepatic impairment. Adjusted dose?
Solution:
Step 1: 10% of 350 = 35 mg
Step 2: New dose = 315 mg
Answer: 315 mg/day
Explanation: Dose reduction.

Problem 435: A patient's 500 mg dose is decreased by 25% for renal impairment. Adjusted dose?
Solution:
Step 1: 25% of 500 = 125 mg
Step 2: New dose = 375 mg
Answer: 375 mg/day
Explanation: Reduce dose.

Problem 436: Dose is 200 mg, reduce by 20% for elderly patient. New dose?
Solution:
Step 1: 20% of 200 = 40 mg
Step 2: New dose = 160 mg
Answer: 160 mg/day
Explanation: Adjust dose.

Problem 437: A 600 mg dose reduced by 15% for hepatic function. What is new dose?
Solution:
Step 1: 15% of 600 = 90 mg
Step 2: New dose = 510 mg
Answer: 510 mg/day
Explanation: Dose reduction.

Problem 438: Patient requires 450 mg, reduce dose by 35%. New dose?
Solution:
Step 1: 35% of 450 = 157.5 mg
Step 2: New dose = 292.5 mg
Answer: 292.5 mg/day
Explanation: Adjust dose.

Problem 439: A dose of 400 mg is decreased by 25% for renal impairment. What is adjusted dose?
Solution:
Step 1: 25% of 400 = 100 mg
Step 2: New dose = 300 mg
Answer: 300 mg/day
Explanation: Dose adjustment.

Problem 440: Dose is 150 mg reduced by 10% for age. New dose?
Solution:
Step 1: 10% of 150 = 15 mg
Step 2: New dose = 135 mg
Answer: 135 mg/day
Explanation: Dose reduction.

Problem 441: A 500 mg dose is reduced by 30%. Adjusted dose?
Solution:
Step 1: 30% of 500 = 150 mg
Step 2: New dose = 350 mg
Answer: 350 mg/day
Explanation: Dose adjustment.

Problem 442: Patient takes 300 mg daily, reduce dose by 20%. New dose?
Solution:
Step 1: 20% of 300 = 60 mg
Step 2: New dose = 240 mg
Answer: 240 mg/day
Explanation: Dose reduction.

Problem 443: Dose of 250 mg reduced by 15%. New dose?
Solution:
Step 1: 15% of 250 = 37.5 mg
Step 2: New dose = 212.5 mg
Answer: 212.5 mg/day
Explanation: Adjust dose.

Problem 444: Patient's dose is 600 mg, reduced by 25%. Adjusted dose?
Solution:
Step 1: 25% of 600 = 150 mg
Step 2: New dose = 450 mg
Answer: 450 mg/day
Explanation: Dose adjustment.

Problem 445: Dose is 400 mg reduced by 10%. New dose?
Solution:
Step 1: 10% of 400 = 40 mg
Step 2: New dose = 360 mg
Answer: 360 mg/day
Explanation: Dose reduction.

Problem 446: A patient takes 350 mg daily, reduce dose by 30%. New dose?
Solution:
Step 1: 30% of 350 = 105 mg
Step 2: New dose = 245 mg
Answer: 245 mg/day
Explanation: Adjust dose.

Problem 447: Dose of 150 mg is reduced by 20%. Adjusted dose?
Solution:
Step 1: 20% of 150 = 30 mg
Step 2: New dose = 120 mg
Answer: 120 mg/day
Explanation: Dose reduction.

Problem 448: Patient requires 500 mg, reduced by 35%. New dose?
Solution:
Step 1: 35% of 500 = 175 mg
Step 2: New dose = 325 mg
Answer: 325 mg/day
Explanation: Dose adjustment.

Problem 449: Dose is 600 mg reduced by 15%. What is new dose?
Solution:
Step 1: 15% of 600 = 90 mg
Step 2: New dose = 510 mg
Answer: 510 mg/day
Explanation: Dose reduction.

Problem 450: A patient takes 400 mg daily, reduced by 25%. Calculate new dose.
Solution:
Step 1: 25% of 400 = 100 mg
Step 2: New dose = 300 mg
Answer: 300 mg/day
Explanation: Adjust dose.

Category 11: Renal & Hepatic Impairment Calculations

Problem 451: A patient with normal kidney function takes 500 mg daily. For moderate renal impairment, dose is reduced by 50%. What is the adjusted dose?
Solution:
Step 1: 50% of 500 mg = 250 mg
Step 2: Adjusted dose = 500 - 250 = 250 mg
Answer: 250 mg/day
Explanation: Reduce dose by half for moderate renal impairment.

Problem 452: A drug is normally dosed 100 mg every 12 hours. Patient's CrCl is 25 mL/min, requiring 40% dose reduction. What is the new dose?
Solution:
Step 1: 40% of 100 = 40 mg
Step 2: New dose = 100 - 40 = 60 mg every 12 hours
Answer: 60 mg every 12 hours
Explanation: Dose adjusted based on creatinine clearance.

Problem 453: A 70 kg patient has CrCl 35 mL/min. Standard dose is 10 mg/kg/day. Reduce dose by 30% for renal impairment. What is adjusted daily dose?
Solution:
Step 1: Standard dose = 10 × 70 = 700 mg
Step 2: 30% reduction = 0.3 × 700 = 210 mg
Step 3: Adjusted dose = 700 - 210 = 490 mg
Answer: 490 mg/day
Explanation: Adjust dose per renal function.

Problem 454: Patient with hepatic impairment requires dose reduction by 35% from 400 mg. Calculate new dose.
Solution:
Step 1: 35% of 400 = 140 mg
Step 2: New dose = 400 - 140 = 260 mg
Answer: 260 mg/day
Explanation: Reduce dose due to liver impairment.

Problem 455: A patient's usual dose is 300 mg daily. Creatinine clearance is 20 mL/min, requiring 50% dose reduction. What is the adjusted dose?
Solution:
Step 1: 50% of 300 = 150 mg
Step 2: New dose = 300 - 150 = 150 mg
Answer: 150 mg/day
Explanation: Dose adjusted for severe renal impairment.

Problem 456: A drug with standard dose 600 mg/day requires 25% dose reduction for moderate hepatic impairment. What is the new dose?
Solution:
Step 1: 25% of 600 = 150 mg
Step 2: Adjusted dose = 600 - 150 = 450 mg
Answer: 450 mg/day
Explanation: Adjust dose for liver impairment.

Problem 457: Patient has CrCl of 45 mL/min. Standard dose 200 mg every 8 hours reduced by 20%. Calculate adjusted dose.
Solution:
Step 1: 20% of 200 = 40 mg

Step 2: New dose = 200 - 40 = 160 mg every 8 hours
Answer: 160 mg every 8 hours
Explanation: Dose adjustment for renal function.

Problem 458: Hepatic impairment requires 40% reduction of a 500 mg daily dose. Calculate new dose.
Solution:
Step 1: 40% of 500 = 200 mg
Step 2: New dose = 500 - 200 = 300 mg
Answer: 300 mg/day
Explanation: Reduce dose for liver impairment.

Problem 459: Patient's normal dose is 250 mg every 12 hours. With CrCl 30 mL/min, reduce dose by 30%. Calculate new dose.
Solution:
Step 1: 30% of 250 = 75 mg
Step 2: New dose = 250 - 75 = 175 mg every 12 hours
Answer: 175 mg every 12 hours
Explanation: Adjust dose based on kidney function.

Problem 460: Hepatic impairment requires 15% reduction of a 400 mg dose. What is the adjusted dose?
Solution:
Step 1: 15% of 400 = 60 mg
Step 2: Adjusted dose = 400 - 60 = 340 mg
Answer: 340 mg
Explanation: Adjust dose accordingly.

Problem 461: CrCl is 25 mL/min; usual dose 600 mg/day is reduced by 50%. Calculate adjusted dose.

234

Solution:
Step 1: 50% of 600 = 300 mg
Step 2: New dose = 300 mg
Answer: 300 mg/day
Explanation: Dose halved for severe renal impairment.

Problem 462: Hepatic impairment requires a 20% dose reduction from 450 mg. What is the new dose?
Solution:
Step 1: 20% of 450 = 90 mg
Step 2: Adjusted dose = 450 - 90 = 360 mg
Answer: 360 mg
Explanation: Dose reduced for liver function.

Problem 463: CrCl 40 mL/min requires 30% dose reduction of 400 mg every 12 hours. Calculate adjusted dose.
Solution:
Step 1: 30% of 400 = 120 mg
Step 2: New dose = 400 - 120 = 280 mg every 12 hours
Answer: 280 mg every 12 hours
Explanation: Adjust dose for kidney impairment.

Problem 464: Hepatic impairment requires 35% reduction of 500 mg dose. Calculate adjusted dose.
Solution:
Step 1: 35% of 500 = 175 mg
Step 2: New dose = 500 - 175 = 325 mg
Answer: 325 mg
Explanation: Reduce dose.

Problem 465: CrCl 20 mL/min requires 60% dose reduction of 300 mg daily dose. Calculate adjusted dose.
Solution:
Step 1: 60% of 300 = 180 mg
Step 2: New dose = 120 mg
Answer: 120 mg/day
Explanation: Significant dose reduction for severe renal impairment.

Problem 466: Hepatic impairment requires a 25% dose reduction of 400 mg daily. What is the adjusted dose?
Solution:
Step 1: 25% of 400 = 100 mg
Step 2: New dose = 300 mg
Answer: 300 mg/day
Explanation: Dose reduced for liver impairment.

Problem 467: CrCl 50 mL/min requires 20% reduction of 500 mg every 8 hours. Calculate adjusted dose.
Solution:
Step 1: 20% of 500 = 100 mg
Step 2: New dose = 400 mg every 8 hours
Answer: 400 mg every 8 hours
Explanation: Adjust dose for mild renal impairment.

Problem 468: Hepatic impairment requires 10% dose reduction of 350 mg. What is new dose?
Solution:
Step 1: 10% of 350 = 35 mg
Step 2: New dose = 315 mg
Answer: 315 mg
Explanation: Minor dose adjustment.

Problem 469: Patient has CrCl 15 mL/min. Dose 300 mg is reduced by 70%. Calculate new dose.
Solution:
Step 1: 70% of 300 = 210 mg
Step 2: New dose = 90 mg
Answer: 90 mg
Explanation: Large dose reduction for severe impairment.

Problem 470: Hepatic impairment requires 30% dose reduction of 600 mg daily. Adjusted dose?
Solution:
Step 1: 30% of 600 = 180 mg
Step 2: New dose = 420 mg
Answer: 420 mg
Explanation: Dose adjustment.

Problem 471: CrCl 35 mL/min requires 40% reduction of 400 mg daily. New dose?
Solution:
Step 1: 40% of 400 = 160 mg
Step 2: New dose = 240 mg
Answer: 240 mg
Explanation: Adjust dose for renal function.

Problem 472: Hepatic impairment requires 20% reduction of 450 mg. Adjusted dose?
Solution:
Step 1: 20% of 450 = 90 mg
Step 2: New dose = 360 mg

Answer: 360 mg
Explanation: Dose adjustment.

Problem 473: CrCl 60 mL/min requires 15% dose reduction of 500 mg daily. Calculate new dose.
Solution:
Step 1: 15% of 500 = 75 mg
Step 2: New dose = 425 mg
Answer: 425 mg
Explanation: Mild reduction for moderate impairment.

Problem 474: Hepatic impairment requires 45% reduction of 400 mg dose. New dose?
Solution:
Step 1: 45% of 400 = 180 mg
Step 2: New dose = 220 mg
Answer: 220 mg
Explanation: Significant reduction.

Problem 475: Patient with CrCl 25 mL/min requires 55% dose reduction of 600 mg daily. New dose?
Solution:
Step 1: 55% of 600 = 330 mg
Step 2: New dose = 270 mg
Answer: 270 mg
Explanation: Large dose reduction.

Problem 476: Hepatic impairment requires 10% dose reduction of 700 mg. Adjusted dose?
Solution:

Step 1: 10% of 700 = 70 mg
Step 2: New dose = 630 mg
Answer: 630 mg
Explanation: Minor adjustment.

Problem 477: CrCl 40 mL/min requires 25% dose reduction of 450 mg every 12 hours. New dose?
Solution:
Step 1: 25% of 450 = 112.5 mg
Step 2: New dose = 337.5 mg every 12 hours
Answer: 337.5 mg every 12 hours
Explanation: Adjust dose for kidney function.

Problem 478: Hepatic impairment requires 30% dose reduction of 500 mg daily. New dose?
Solution:
Step 1: 30% of 500 = 150 mg
Step 2: New dose = 350 mg
Answer: 350 mg
Explanation: Dose reduction.

Problem 479: Patient with CrCl 20 mL/min requires 60% dose reduction of 400 mg daily. Adjusted dose?
Solution:
Step 1: 60% of 400 = 240 mg
Step 2: New dose = 160 mg
Answer: 160 mg
Explanation: Large reduction.

Problem 480: Hepatic impairment requires 50% dose reduction of 300 mg. New dose?
Solution:
Step 1: 50% of 300 = 150 mg
Step 2: New dose = 150 mg
Answer: 150 mg
Explanation: Significant dose reduction.

Problem 481: CrCl 55 mL/min requires 20% dose reduction of 600 mg daily. New dose?
Solution:
Step 1: 20% of 600 = 120 mg
Step 2: New dose = 480 mg
Answer: 480 mg
Explanation: Mild reduction.

Problem 482: Hepatic impairment requires 40% dose reduction of 400 mg daily. New dose?
Solution:
Step 1: 40% of 400 = 160 mg
Step 2: New dose = 240 mg
Answer: 240 mg
Explanation: Adjust dose.

Problem 483: Patient with CrCl 30 mL/min requires 35% dose reduction of 500 mg every 12 hours. New dose?
Solution:
Step 1: 35% of 500 = 175 mg
Step 2: New dose = 325 mg every 12 hours
Answer: 325 mg every 12 hours
Explanation: Adjust dose.

Problem 484: Hepatic impairment requires 15% dose reduction of 700 mg. New dose?
Solution:
Step 1: 15% of 700 = 105 mg
Step 2: New dose = 595 mg
Answer: 595 mg
Explanation: Adjust dose.

Problem 485: CrCl 25 mL/min requires 45% dose reduction of 400 mg daily. New dose?
Solution:
Step 1: 45% of 400 = 180 mg
Step 2: New dose = 220 mg
Answer: 220 mg
Explanation: Adjust dose.

Problem 486: Hepatic impairment requires 30% dose reduction of 600 mg. New dose?
Solution:
Step 1: 30% of 600 = 180 mg
Step 2: New dose = 420 mg
Answer: 420 mg
Explanation: Adjust dose.

Problem 487: Patient with CrCl 50 mL/min requires 20% dose reduction of 300 mg daily. New dose?
Solution:
Step 1: 20% of 300 = 60 mg
Step 2: New dose = 240 mg

Answer: 240 mg
Explanation: Adjust dose.

Problem 488: Hepatic impairment requires 35% dose reduction of 500 mg daily. New dose?
Solution:
Step 1: 35% of 500 = 175 mg
Step 2: New dose = 325 mg
Answer: 325 mg
Explanation: Dose adjustment.

Problem 489: Patient with CrCl 40 mL/min requires 25% dose reduction of 600 mg daily. New dose?
Solution:
Step 1: 25% of 600 = 150 mg
Step 2: New dose = 450 mg
Answer: 450 mg
Explanation: Dose adjustment.

Problem 490: Hepatic impairment requires 10% dose reduction of 400 mg. New dose?
Solution:
Step 1: 10% of 400 = 40 mg
Step 2: New dose = 360 mg
Answer: 360 mg
Explanation: Dose adjustment.

Problem 491: CrCl 20 mL/min requires 50% dose reduction of 300 mg daily. New dose?
Solution:

Step 1: 50% of 300 = 150 mg
Step 2: New dose = 150 mg
Answer: 150 mg
Explanation: Dose adjustment.

Problem 492: Hepatic impairment requires 45% dose reduction of 700 mg. New dose?
Solution:
Step 1: 45% of 700 = 315 mg
Step 2: New dose = 385 mg
Answer: 385 mg
Explanation: Dose adjustment.

Problem 493: Patient with CrCl 60 mL/min requires 15% dose reduction of 500 mg daily. New dose?
Solution:
Step 1: 15% of 500 = 75 mg
Step 2: New dose = 425 mg
Answer: 425 mg
Explanation: Dose adjustment.

Problem 494: Hepatic impairment requires 25% dose reduction of 600 mg. New dose?
Solution:
Step 1: 25% of 600 = 150 mg
Step 2: New dose = 450 mg
Answer: 450 mg
Explanation: Dose adjustment.

Problem 495: Patient with CrCl 35 mL/min requires 35% dose reduction of 400 mg daily. New dose?
Solution:
Step 1: 35% of 400 = 140 mg
Step 2: New dose = 260 mg
Answer: 260 mg
Explanation: Dose adjustment.

Problem 496: Hepatic impairment requires 30% dose reduction of 500 mg daily. New dose?
Solution:
Step 1: 30% of 500 = 150 mg
Step 2: New dose = 350 mg
Answer: 350 mg
Explanation: Dose adjustment.

Problem 497: Patient with CrCl 50 mL/min requires 20% dose reduction of 600 mg daily. New dose?
Solution:
Step 1: 20% of 600 = 120 mg
Step 2: New dose = 480 mg
Answer: 480 mg
Explanation: Dose adjustment.

Problem 498: Hepatic impairment requires 15% dose reduction of 400 mg. New dose?
Solution:
Step 1: 15% of 400 = 60 mg
Step 2: New dose = 340 mg
Answer: 340 mg
Explanation: Dose adjustment.

244

Problem 499: Patient with CrCl 25 mL/min requires 40% dose reduction of 300 mg daily. New dose?
Solution:
Step 1: 40% of 300 = 120 mg
Step 2: New dose = 180 mg
Answer: 180 mg
Explanation: Dose adjustment.

Problem 500: Hepatic impairment requires 20% dose reduction of 600 mg. New dose?
Solution:
Step 1: 20% of 600 = 120 mg
Step 2: New dose = 480 mg
Answer: 480 mg
Explanation: Dose adjustment.

Appendix A: Quick Reference Guide

The clinical world moves fast, and you need information at your fingertips when calculations matter most. This reference guide becomes your constant companion—a tool that transforms scattered knowledge into organized, accessible resources you can trust during high-pressure situations. Think of this as your mathematical safety net, designed to catch errors before they reach patients and support your confidence when stakes are highest.

Healthcare professionals who succeed develop systematic approaches to information management. They create reliable reference systems that reduce cognitive load during complex calculations while maintaining accuracy standards that protect patient safety. This guide provides exactly that framework—organizing essential information in formats that work efficiently during real clinical practice.

Common Conversion Factors You'll Use Daily

Weight Conversions That Save Lives

Every weight conversion you perform affects medication dosing, and small errors multiply into dangerous consequences. Master these conversions until they become automatic responses rather than conscious calculations.

The fundamental relationship: **1 kilogram equals 2.2 pounds**. This conversion appears in virtually every weight-based medication calculation you perform throughout your career. When converting pounds to kilograms, divide by 2.2. When converting kilograms to pounds, multiply by 2.2.

Common weight conversions you'll encounter frequently:

- 110 pounds = 50 kg (110 ÷ 2.2)
- 154 pounds = 70 kg (154 ÷ 2.2)
- 176 pounds = 80 kg (176 ÷ 2.2)

- 25 kg = 55 pounds (25 × 2.2)
- 30 kg = 66 pounds (30 × 2.2)

Round weights to the nearest tenth of a kilogram for most calculations. This precision level provides accuracy without unnecessary complexity for routine clinical calculations.

Metric System Mastery

The metric system's logical structure makes conversions predictable once you understand the patterns. Each prefix represents a specific power of ten relationship that creates consistent conversion rules across all measurements.

Within weight measurements: 1 kilogram = 1,000 grams = 1,000,000 milligrams = 1,000,000,000 micrograms. Moving from larger to smaller units requires multiplication (moving decimal points right). Moving from smaller to larger units requires division (moving decimal points left).

Volume relationships follow identical patterns: 1 liter = 1,000 milliliters. For practical nursing purposes, 1 milliliter equals 1 cubic centimeter, though many institutions prefer mL notation for clarity and safety.

Household Measurements for Patient Education

Patients use household measurements at home, making these conversions essential for discharge planning and medication compliance. These approximations provide sufficient accuracy for most home administration while offering familiar reference points.

Standard household equivalents include: 1 teaspoon = 5 mL, 1 tablespoon = 15 mL, 1 fluid ounce = 30 mL, 1 cup = 240 mL. These conversions help you translate precise medical measurements into practical home administration instructions.

Time Conversions for Infusion Calculations

IV calculations frequently require time unit conversions between minutes, hours, and days. Master these relationships: 1 hour = 60 minutes, 1 day = 24 hours, 1 day = 1,440 minutes.

These conversions appear in flow rate calculations, medication timing, and protocol adjustments. Practice converting between units until these relationships become automatic responses during complex calculations.

Formula Summary Cards for Quick Reference

The Universal Dimensional Analysis Setup

Dimensional analysis provides the most reliable method for complex medication calculations because it builds verification into the calculation process. The basic structure remains constant regardless of calculation complexity.

Starting amount × (conversion factor 1) × (conversion factor 2) × ... = final answer

Each conversion factor represents equivalent amounts expressed in different units. Arrange factors so unwanted units cancel, leaving only desired units in the final answer. This visual confirmation prevents setup errors that cause calculation mistakes.

Essential Formulas for Daily Practice

Basic medication calculation formula: Desired dose ÷ Available dose × Vehicle = Amount to give

This formula works efficiently for straightforward calculations where units are already compatible. Use it for simple tablet calculations and liquid medications when no conversions are required.

IV flow rate formula: Total volume ÷ Time in hours = mL/hr

Program this rate into infusion pumps for controlled delivery. This formula applies to maintenance fluids, intermittent medications, and continuous infusions.

Gravity infusion formula: (Total volume × Drop factor) ÷ Time in minutes = Drops per minute

Use this calculation when infusion pumps aren't available. Remember that microdrip tubing (60 drops/mL) simplifies calculations because mL/hr equals drops/minute.

Weight-based dosing formula: mg/kg × Weight in kg = Total dose

This calculation determines medication amounts based on patient weight. Divide by dosing frequency if the dose represents total daily amount rather than individual dose.

Concentration calculation formula: Amount of medication ÷ Volume of solution = Concentration

Use this formula to determine medication concentrations for continuous infusions and to verify preparation accuracy.

Abbreviation Safety List

Approved Abbreviations That Prevent Errors

Healthcare abbreviations reduce documentation time while maintaining communication clarity, but only when used correctly and consistently. Learn approved abbreviations and avoid dangerous alternatives that cause medication errors.

Safe medication abbreviations include: mg (milligrams), mL (milliliters), kg (kilograms), hr (hours), min (minutes), IV (intravenous), PO (by mouth), IM (intramuscular), SubQ (subcutaneous).

Dangerous Abbreviations to Avoid

The Joint Commission maintains a "Do Not Use" list of abbreviations that cause frequent medication errors. These abbreviations create confusion that leads to wrong doses, wrong medications, or wrong routes.

Never use: U or u (for units - write "units"), IU (for international units - write "international units"), Q.D. or QD (for daily - write "daily"), Q.O.D. or QOD (for every other day - write "every other day").

Decimal point errors prove particularly dangerous: Always write 0.5 mg (not .5 mg) and 5 mg (not 5.0 mg unless trailing zero adds necessary clarity).

Route Abbreviations for Safe Administration

Route abbreviations specify how medications should be given, preventing dangerous administration errors. Use standard abbreviations consistently: PO (by mouth), IV (intravenous), IM (intramuscular), SubQ (subcutaneous), SL (sublingual), PR (per rectum), OD (right eye), OS (left eye), OU (both eyes).

Frequency Abbreviations for Accurate Timing

Timing abbreviations communicate medication schedules clearly: BID (twice daily), TID (three times daily), QID (four times daily), Q4H (every 4 hours), Q6H (every 6 hours), Q8H (every 8 hours), Q12H (every 12 hours), PRN (as needed).

High-Alert Medication List

Medications That Demand Extra Vigilance

High-alert medications can cause severe patient harm when used incorrectly, making them priority targets for error prevention strategies. These medications require independent double-checking, standardized concentrations, and enhanced monitoring protocols.

Insulin preparations top most high-alert lists because dosing errors cause rapid, severe hypoglycemia that can result in coma or death. All insulin calculations require independent verification by two qualified staff members. Use only insulin syringes for insulin administration, and always verify concentration matches syringe calibration.

Heparin and anticoagulants cause bleeding complications when dosed incorrectly. Therapeutic heparin protocols specify exact dosing parameters and monitoring requirements. Flush solutions use much lower concentrations than therapeutic doses—never confuse these preparations.

Vasoactive medications (dopamine, norepinephrine, epinephrine) directly affect heart function and blood pressure. Small concentration changes produce dramatic physiologic effects. These medications require continuous monitoring and precise calculation accuracy.

Chemotherapy agents destroy both cancer cells and normal cells, creating narrow therapeutic windows with severe toxicity potential. Most chemotherapy calculations require pharmacist verification and oncology nurse administration.

Narcotics and sedatives depress respiratory function, especially when combined with other central nervous system depressants. Calculate doses carefully and monitor patients continuously, particularly during initial administration.

Electrolyte solutions (potassium, magnesium, calcium) affect cardiac rhythm and nerve function. Concentrated solutions require controlled infusion rates and cardiac monitoring during administration.

Case Example: High-Alert Medication Protocol

Margaret Foster, a 68-year-old woman with atrial fibrillation, needs therapeutic heparin after cardiac catheterization. She weighs 75 kg with normal kidney function.

Protocol requirements: Initial bolus 80 units/kg IV push, followed by continuous infusion at 18 units/kg/hr. PTT monitoring every 6 hours with dose adjustments per protocol table.

Independent verification process: Both nurses calculate independently— Nurse 1: Bolus = 75 kg × 80 units/kg = 6,000 units Infusion = 75 kg × 18 units/kg/hr = 1,350 units/hr

Nurse 2: Same calculations using different method— Bolus = 80 × 75 = 6,000 units ✓ Infusion = 18 × 75 = 1,350 units/hr ✓

Concentration calculations: Using 25,000 units in 250 mL (100 units/mL) Bolus volume: 6,000 units ÷ 5,000 units/mL = 1.2 mL IV push Infusion rate: 1,350 units/hr ÷ 100 units/mL = 13.5 mL/hr

Both nurses verify calculations, check concentrations, and document independent verification before administration.

Rounding Rules by Medication Type

Oral Medications Rounding Guidelines

Tablet calculations often yield decimal results that require practical rounding for administration. Round to the nearest half-tablet when tablets are scored and can be split safely. Round to the nearest whole tablet when tablets cannot be split.

Liquid oral medications round to the nearest tenth of a milliliter when using oral syringes (0.1 mL precision). Round to the nearest half-milliliter when using measuring cups or less precise devices.

Injectable Medication Precision Requirements

Injectable medications demand higher precision than oral medications because of immediate absorption and inability to retrieve doses once administered. Round subcutaneous and intramuscular injections to the nearest hundredth (0.01 mL) when using 1 mL syringes. Round to the nearest tenth (0.1 mL) when using larger syringes.

Insulin calculations round to the nearest unit when using insulin syringes calibrated for U-100 insulin. Higher concentration insulins may require different rounding protocols—verify with pharmacy before administration.

IV Medication Rounding Protocols

Infusion pump programming typically accepts tenths of mL/hr, making this the standard rounding precision for most IV calculations. Critical care medications may require hundredths precision for very low flow rates.

Pediatric IV calculations often require greater precision due to smaller patient size and narrower therapeutic windows. Follow institutional protocols for pediatric-specific rounding requirements.

Case Example: Rounding Decision Process

David Chen, a 55-year-old man, needs acetaminophen for post-operative pain. The order specifies 650 mg every 6 hours. Available tablets contain 325 mg each.

Calculation: 650 mg ÷ 325 mg/tablet = 2 tablets exactly

This calculation yields a whole number, requiring no rounding decisions. Give 2 tablets per dose.

Alternative scenario: Same patient needs 500 mg acetaminophen with 325 mg tablets available.

Calculation: 500 mg ÷ 325 mg/tablet = 1.54 tablets

Since 325 mg tablets are scored and can be split safely, round to 1.5 tablets (half-tablet precision). This provides 487.5 mg—close to the prescribed 500 mg and within acceptable variance.

Documentation: Record "acetaminophen 1.5 tablets (487.5 mg) given PO for pain" to show exact amount administered.

Reference Foundation: Building Clinical Confidence

This quick reference guide transforms scattered information into organized, accessible tools that support accurate calculations throughout your nursing career. These conversion factors, formulas, and safety guidelines become second nature through repeated use, building the mathematical confidence you need for complex clinical situations.

Your ability to access accurate information quickly distinguishes competent practitioners from those who struggle with routine calculations. Keep these references easily accessible during clinical practice, and refer to them whenever uncertainty arises. Consistent use builds familiarity that eventually makes these tools automatic parts of your calculation process.

The safety protocols and high-alert medication guidelines protect both patients and practitioners by establishing systematic approaches to error-prone situations. Follow these guidelines consistently, and encourage colleagues to maintain the same standards for collaborative patient safety.

Key Takeaways for Quick Reference Success

- Common conversion factors become automatic responses through regular practice and consistent application
- Formula summary cards provide systematic approaches that work reliably under pressure and time constraints
- Abbreviation safety knowledge prevents communication errors that lead to medication administration mistakes
- High-alert medication protocols require extra vigilance and independent verification to prevent serious patient harm
- Rounding rules vary by medication type and administration route, requiring careful attention to precision requirements

Appendix B: Additional Practice by Topic

Practice transforms theoretical knowledge into clinical competence. You need deliberate, focused practice that builds skills systematically while addressing individual learning needs. This appendix provides targeted exercises designed to strengthen specific calculation areas while building overall mathematical confidence for patient care responsibilities.

The practice problems here go beyond simple repetition—they're crafted to address common error patterns, build pattern recognition skills, and develop the clinical reasoning that distinguishes expert practitioners from those who merely follow algorithms. Each problem set includes progressive difficulty levels that challenge you appropriately while building confidence through successful problem-solving experiences.

Foundation Skills Building Exercises

Basic Mathematical Operations for Healthcare

Healthcare calculations require rock-solid basic math skills because errors in fundamental operations propagate through complex problems, creating dangerous patient safety issues. These exercises rebuild mathematical confidence while addressing specific healthcare applications.

Fraction Operations in Medical Context

Practice converting between fractions and decimals using medication-relevant examples. Start with simple conversions: $1/4 = 0.25$, $1/2 = 0.5$, $3/4 = 0.75$. These relationships appear constantly in tablet splitting calculations and liquid medication measurements.

Work through practical problems: A patient needs 3/4 of a 20 mg tablet. Calculate the dose in mg: $3/4 \times 20$ mg $= 15$ mg. A liquid medication contains 2/3 of its original concentration after dilution. If the original concentration was 300 mg/5 mL, what's the new concentration? 2/3 × 300 mg = 200 mg per 5 mL.

Decimal Precision for Patient Safety

Decimal point errors cause more medication mistakes than any other mathematical error. Practice reading decimals aloud correctly: 0.125 mg is "zero point one two five milligrams," never "point one twenty-five." This precision prevents confusion between 0.125 mg and 125 mg—a potentially fatal thousand-fold error.

Calculate decimal operations systematically: 2.5 mg + 1.25 mg = 3.75 mg. When multiplying decimals, count total decimal places in both numbers: 0.5 × 2.25 = 1.125 (one decimal place plus two decimal places equals three decimal places in the answer).

Percentage Applications for Clinical Practice

Many medication concentrations express as percentages, requiring conversion skills for accurate calculations. A 1% solution contains 1 gram of medication per 100 mL of solution. Calculate how many milligrams per mL this represents: 1 gram = 1,000 mg, so 1,000 mg ÷ 100 mL = 10 mg/mL.

Practice percentage-to-decimal conversions: 0.9% sodium chloride = 0.009, 5% dextrose = 0.05, 20% mannitol = 0.20. These conversions help you work with various solution concentrations in clinical practice.

Weight-Based Dosing Practice Sets

Pediatric Weight-Based Calculations

Pediatric dosing requires exceptional precision because children have narrow therapeutic windows and limited ability to communicate adverse effects. These practice problems build systematic approaches to safe pediatric calculations.

Case-Based Practice Problem Set One

Emma Johnson, age 4, weighs 18 kg and needs amoxicillin for strep throat. The prescribed dose is 40 mg/kg/day divided into three doses. Available suspension contains 250 mg per 5 mL.

Calculate step-by-step: Daily dose = 18 kg × 40 mg/kg/day = 720 mg/day. Individual dose = 720 mg/day ÷ 3 doses = 240 mg per dose. Volume per dose = 240 mg × (5 mL/250 mg) = 4.8 mL per dose.

Verify your calculation: 4.8 mL × (250 mg/5 mL) = 240 mg √. Daily volume = 4.8 mL × 3 doses = 14.4 mL total daily.

Convert to household measurements for family: 4.8 mL ÷ 5 mL per teaspoon = 0.96 teaspoons ≈ 1 teaspoon per dose.

Adult Weight-Based Protocol Practice

Many adult medications use weight-based dosing, particularly in critical care and emergency medicine. These problems develop skills for adult weight-based calculations while considering clinical monitoring requirements.

Case-Based Practice Problem Set Two

Robert Martinez, a 35-year-old man weighing 175 pounds, needs heparin for pulmonary embolism treatment. The protocol specifies: bolus dose 80 units/kg IV push, then continuous infusion at 18 units/kg/hr.

Convert weight: 175 pounds ÷ 2.2 = 79.5 kg (round to 80 kg for calculation simplicity). Calculate bolus: 80 kg × 80 units/kg = 6,400 units IV push. Calculate infusion rate: 80 kg × 18 units/kg/hr = 1,440 units/hr.

Determine volume calculations: Using 5,000 units/mL for bolus— 6,400 units ÷ 5,000 units/mL = 1.28 mL IV push. Using 25,000 units in 250 mL for infusion (100 units/mL)—1,440 units/hr ÷ 100 units/mL = 14.4 mL/hr.

IV Flow Rate Calculation Drills

Pump Programming Scenarios

Modern nursing requires fluency with infusion pump calculations because most IV medications deliver through controlled pump systems. These drills build speed and accuracy with pump-related calculations.

Time-Based Calculation Series

Calculate infusion completion times for care planning purposes. A 1,000 mL IV bag infuses at 125 mL/hr. How long will it take to complete? 1,000 mL ÷ 125 mL/hr = 8 hours. If started at 0800, completion time is 1600 (4:00 PM).

Practice with varying rates and volumes: 250 mL antibiotic infuses at 100 mL/hr—completion time is 2.5 hours. 500 mL blood transfusion infuses at 75 mL/hr—completion time is 6.67 hours (approximately 6 hours 40 minutes).

Rate Adjustment Calculations

Clinical situations often require infusion rate changes to maintain therapeutic levels or correct timing delays. Practice calculating new rates when schedules change.

Case-Based Practice Problem Set Three

Patricia Williams receives 1,500 mL lactated Ringer's solution that should complete in 12 hours. After 6 hours, only 600 mL has infused due to IV infiltration and restart delays. Calculate the new rate needed to finish on time.

Remaining volume: 1,500 mL - 600 mL = 900 mL. Remaining time: 12 hours - 6 hours = 6 hours. New rate: 900 mL ÷ 6 hours = 150 mL/hr.

Verify this rate is safe and appropriate for the patient's condition before implementing. Some rate increases may exceed safe limits or patient tolerance.

Concentration and Dilution Problems

Solution Preparation Calculations

Critical care nursing often requires medication dilution calculations for continuous infusions and specialized preparations. These problems develop skills for safe solution preparation.

Stock Solution Dilution Practice

Calculate how to prepare desired concentrations from available stock solutions. You need 100 mL of 0.5% lidocaine solution. Available stock contains 2% lidocaine. How much stock solution and diluent do you need?

Use the dilution formula: $C_1 \times V_1 = C_2 \times V_2$ where C_1 = stock concentration, V_1 = stock volume needed, C_2 = desired concentration, V_2 = desired final volume.

$2\% \times V_1 = 0.5\% \times 100$ mL, so $V_1 = (0.5 \times 100) \div 2 = 25$ mL of stock solution. Diluent needed: 100 mL - 25 mL = 75 mL sterile water.

Critical Care Drip Calculations

Vasoactive medications require precise concentration calculations for accurate dosing. Practice preparing standard concentrations used in critical care units.

Case-Based Practice Problem Set Four

Michael Thompson, weighing 70 kg, needs dopamine at 10 mcg/kg/min. Your unit uses standard concentration of 400 mg dopamine in 250 mL D5W.

Calculate hourly dose: 70 kg × 10 mcg/kg/min × 60 min/hr = 42,000 mcg/hr = 42 mg/hr. Calculate concentration: 400 mg ÷ 250 mL = 1.6 mg/mL. Calculate infusion rate: 42 mg/hr ÷ 1.6 mg/mL = 26.25 mL/hr.

Program pump for 26.3 mL/hr (rounded to nearest tenth). Monitor patient response and adjust per protocol.

Error Recognition and Prevention Exercises

Common Error Pattern Identification

Learning to recognize calculation errors before they reach patients builds an essential safety skill. These exercises train your ability to spot mistakes in your own work and others' calculations.

Decimal Point Error Recognition

Practice identifying decimal point errors in medication orders and calculations. A physician orders digoxin 2.5 mg daily for heart failure. Does this dose seem reasonable? Standard digoxin dosing ranges from 0.125-0.25 mg daily. The ordered dose represents a 10-fold error— likely intended as 0.25 mg.

Another example: Insulin calculation yields 50 units for a sliding scale. Typical sliding scale doses range from 2-10 units. This calculation likely contains an error requiring verification before administration.

Unit Confusion Prevention

Different units for similar measurements create frequent calculation errors. Practice converting between units correctly: 1 mg = 1,000 mcg, 1 g = 1,000 mg, 1 kg = 1,000 g.

Case-Based Practice Problem Set Five

A medication order specifies 500 mcg of a drug. Available tablets contain 0.5 mg each. How many tablets should you give?

Convert to common units: 500 mcg = 0.5 mg (500 ÷ 1,000). Calculate tablets needed: 0.5 mg ÷ 0.5 mg/tablet = 1 tablet.

Verify by working backwards: 1 tablet × 0.5 mg/tablet = 0.5 mg = 500 mcg √

Visual Learning Aids and Memory Tools

Conversion Factor Memory Aids

Visual associations help you recall important conversion factors during high-pressure situations. Create mental images that connect numbers with familiar objects or experiences.

Associate 2.2 pounds per kilogram with common objects: a bag of sugar weighs approximately 2.2 pounds (1 kg). Use this reference for quick weight estimation and conversion verification.

Formula Memory Techniques

Develop memorable phrases for essential formulas. For dimensional analysis setup: "Start with what you have, multiply by what converts, end with what you want." This phrase reminds you to begin calculations with the given information and arrange conversion factors to achieve desired units.

Syringe Reading Practice

Visual exercises improve accuracy when reading syringes and measuring devices. Practice with images of various syringe types: 1 mL syringes with 0.01 mL graduations, 3 mL syringes with 0.1 mL graduations, insulin syringes with unit markings.

Case-Based Practice Problem Set Six

Jennifer Kim needs morphine 2.5 mg IV for pain. Available concentration is 10 mg/mL. Calculate volume needed: 2.5 mg ÷ 10 mg/mL = 0.25 mL.

Which syringe provides best accuracy? A 1 mL syringe allows precise 0.25 mL measurement. A 3 mL syringe rounds to 0.3 mL due to graduation limitations. Choose the 1 mL syringe for optimal accuracy.

Progressive Difficulty Challenges

Beginner Level Integration

Combine basic skills into realistic clinical scenarios that challenge your growing competence without overwhelming your confidence. These problems integrate multiple calculation types while maintaining manageable complexity.

Intermediate Clinical Applications

Build on basic skills with problems requiring multiple conversion steps and clinical reasoning. These scenarios mirror real-world complexity while providing sufficient structure for systematic problem-solving.

Advanced Multi-Step Scenarios

Challenge your developing expertise with complex problems requiring integration of multiple calculation methods, clinical judgment, and error prevention strategies. These problems prepare you for the most challenging clinical situations you'll encounter.

Case-Based Practice Problem Set Seven

Maria Rodriguez, a 45-year-old woman weighing 65 kg, needs pain management after major surgery. Current orders include: morphine

PCA 1 mg bolus dose with 6-minute lockout, continuous rate 0.5 mg/hr, 4-hour limit 20 mg.

Calculate various parameters: Maximum boluses per hour = 60 minutes ÷ 6-minute lockout = 10 boluses maximum. Maximum hourly dose = (10 boluses × 1 mg) + 0.5 mg continuous = 10.5 mg/hr maximum. Verify 4-hour limit: 20 mg ÷ 4 hours = 5 mg/hr average— lower than maximum hourly rate, so the 4-hour limit is the controlling factor.

Monitor patient's actual usage patterns and assess pain relief effectiveness. Adjust parameters per physician orders and institutional protocols.

Skill Building: Your Path to Calculation Mastery

These practice exercises transform theoretical knowledge into practical competence through systematic skill building and progressive challenges. Regular practice with varied problem types builds the pattern recognition and automatic responses you need for safe, confident clinical practice.

Your commitment to deliberate practice distinguishes you as a practitioner serious about calculation accuracy and patient safety. Each problem you solve correctly builds confidence while reinforcing systematic approaches that work reliably under pressure.

The skills you develop through focused practice become tools you rely on throughout your career, enabling you to function confidently in any healthcare environment while maintaining the accuracy standards that protect patient safety.

Key Takeaways for Practice Success

- Foundation skills require regular practice to maintain automatic responses during complex calculations
- Weight-based dosing problems build systematic approaches essential for safe pediatric and critical care practice

- IV flow rate drills develop fluency with pump programming and timing calculations needed for modern nursing practice
- Concentration and dilution problems prepare you for critical care medication preparation responsibilities
- Error recognition exercises build pattern identification skills that prevent mistakes before they reach patients

Appendix C: Clinical Correlation Tables

Clinical practice demands more than isolated calculation skills—you need integrated knowledge that connects mathematical accuracy with patient safety protocols, equipment specifications, and specialty-specific requirements. These correlation tables organize critical information in formats that support real-world decision-making while reinforcing the clinical context that makes calculations meaningful.

Understanding how calculations fit within broader clinical frameworks distinguishes competent practitioners from those who perform calculations mechanically without grasping their therapeutic significance. These tables provide the clinical correlations needed to make informed decisions about medication calculations across diverse healthcare environments.

Specialty-Specific Calculation Requirements

Critical Care Unit Standards

Critical care environments require heightened calculation precision because patients have minimal physiologic reserves and medication errors cause rapid, severe consequences. ICU calculation standards exceed general unit requirements in accuracy, verification protocols, and monitoring intensity.

Vasoactive medication calculations in critical care units follow standardized concentration protocols that reduce complexity while maintaining safety. Most units use predetermined concentrations for common drugs: dopamine 400 mg in 250 mL, norepinephrine 4 mg in 250 mL, epinephrine 1 mg in 250 mL. These standards allow development of calculation shortcuts and dosing tables that improve efficiency during emergencies.

Weight-based dosing calculations require frequent updates as patient conditions change. ICU patients may gain or lose significant fluid weight during stays, affecting medication dosing accuracy. Verify weights daily and recalculate weight-based medications when clinical changes suggest significant weight variations.

Insulin infusion protocols in critical care units typically target glucose ranges of 140-180 mg/dL with hourly monitoring and frequent rate adjustments. These protocols require rapid calculation skills because delayed responses to glucose changes can worsen patient outcomes. Practice insulin protocol calculations until adjustments become automatic responses to glucose trends.

Emergency Department Protocols

Emergency departments demand rapid, accurate calculations for time-critical interventions where delays can mean the difference between life and death. ED calculation protocols prioritize speed while maintaining safety through systematic approaches and verification procedures.

Cardiac arrest calculations require immediate accuracy for medications that must be given within minutes of arrest identification. Standard adult doses include: epinephrine 1 mg IV every 3-5 minutes, amiodarone 300 mg IV for first dose, followed by 150 mg IV for second dose. Pediatric doses calculate as epinephrine 0.01 mg/kg IV, amiodarone 5 mg/kg IV.

Pain management calculations in emergency settings balance rapid relief with safety considerations. Standard protocols include: morphine 0.1 mg/kg IV for adults, fentanyl 1-2 mcg/kg IV for rapid onset, hydromorphone 0.015 mg/kg IV for alternative opioid choice. Pediatric pain dosing typically follows similar mg/kg calculations with maximum dose limits.

Fluid resuscitation calculations for trauma and shock patients require rapid volume determinations based on estimated blood loss and physiologic parameters. Standard protocols include: crystalloid 3:1 replacement ratio for estimated blood loss, initial bolus 20 mL/kg for adults, 10-20 mL/kg for children depending on clinical condition.

Pediatric Unit Considerations

Pediatric calculations require specialized approaches that account for developmental physiology, weight-based dosing precision, and age-appropriate administration techniques. Pediatric units maintain stricter accuracy standards due to children's narrow therapeutic windows and limited ability to communicate adverse effects.

Medication dosing in pediatrics typically calculates per kilogram of body weight rather than using standard adult doses. Common pediatric calculations include: acetaminophen 10-15 mg/kg every 4-6 hours, ibuprofen 5-10 mg/kg every 6-8 hours, amoxicillin 20-40 mg/kg/day divided into appropriate doses.

Volume limitations for pediatric administration affect calculation approaches and medication selection. Oral medications should not exceed 5 mL per dose for infants, 10 mL per dose for toddlers, and 15 mL per dose for school-age children. Injectable volumes must stay within 0.5 mL for infants, 1 mL for toddlers, and 2 mL for older children per injection site.

Oncology Calculation Protocols

Oncology units require specialized calculation skills for chemotherapy agents that have narrow therapeutic windows and severe toxicity potential. These calculations typically use body surface area rather than weight alone and require extensive verification procedures.

Chemotherapy dosing calculations use BSA (body surface area) measured in square meters. Calculate BSA using the formula: BSA = $\sqrt{[(\text{height in cm} \times \text{weight in kg}) \div 3{,}600]}$. Most oncology units use BSA nomograms or electronic calculators to reduce calculation errors and improve efficiency.

Dose modification calculations for chemotherapy account for patient toxicity, organ function, and previous treatment tolerance. Standard modifications include: 25% dose reduction for grade 2 toxicity, 50%

dose reduction for grade 3 toxicity, treatment hold for grade 4 toxicity until resolution to grade 1 or baseline.

Case Example: Specialty-Specific Calculation Application

David Thompson, a 28-year-old man, presents to the emergency department with severe allergic reaction requiring immediate epinephrine. He weighs 80 kg and shows signs of anaphylaxis with respiratory distress and hypotension.

Emergency calculation: Epinephrine dose = 0.01 mg/kg = 0.01 × 80 = 0.8 mg IV push. Available concentration is 1:10,000 (0.1 mg/mL). Volume needed = 0.8 mg ÷ 0.1 mg/mL = 8 mL IV push immediately.

Follow-up calculation: Patient requires epinephrine infusion for refractory hypotension. Standard concentration: 1 mg in 250 mL D5W (4 mcg/mL). Starting dose: 2 mcg/min = 2 mcg/min × 60 min/hr ÷ 4 mcg/mL = 30 mL/hr initial rate.

Clinical correlation: Emergency department protocols require immediate epinephrine administration without delays for complex calculations. Standard dosing tables and pre-calculated concentrations enable rapid response while maintaining dosing accuracy.

Common Medication Concentrations

Standard Critical Care Concentrations

Critical care units use standardized medication concentrations to reduce calculation complexity and improve safety during high-acuity situations. These standards create consistency across units while enabling development of calculation shortcuts and dosing tables.

Vasopressor standard concentrations include dopamine 400 mg or 800 mg in 250 mL, norepinephrine 4 mg or 8 mg in 250 mL, epinephrine 1 mg or 2 mg in 250 mL, phenylephrine 10 mg in 250 mL. These concentrations support weight-based dosing calculations while providing reasonable infusion rates for pump programming.

Sedation medication concentrations follow similar standardization principles: propofol 10 mg/mL (ready-to-use), midazolam 1 mg/mL or 5 mg/mL depending on application, fentanyl 50 mcg/mL, dexmedetomidine 4 mcg/mL. These concentrations balance dose flexibility with calculation simplicity.

Cardiac medication concentrations for specialized applications include amiodarone 1.5 mg/mL for infusions, diltiazem 1 mg/mL for rate control, esmolol 10 mg/mL for short-acting beta-blockade, nitroglycerin 50 mg in 250 mL for afterload reduction.

Emergency Department Standard Preparations

Emergency departments maintain ready-to-use concentrations for time-critical medications where preparation delays can compromise patient outcomes. These concentrations enable immediate administration while maintaining dosing accuracy.

Cardiac arrest medications come in standard concentrations: epinephrine 1 mg in 10 mL prefilled syringes (1:10,000), amiodarone 150 mg in 3 mL prefilled syringes, atropine 1 mg in 10 mL prefilled syringes, lidocaine 100 mg in 5 mL prefilled syringes.

Pain management concentrations for emergency use include morphine 10 mg/mL vials, fentanyl 50 mcg/mL vials, hydromorphone 2 mg/mL vials, ketorolac 30 mg/mL vials. These concentrations support rapid dosing calculations while providing appropriate volumes for administration.

Pediatric Emergency Concentrations

Pediatric emergency medications require specialized concentrations that support weight-based dosing while providing measurable volumes for small patients. Many pediatric medications come in diluted concentrations specifically designed for children.

Pediatric resuscitation medications include epinephrine 1:10,000 (0.1 mg/mL) for cardiac arrest, atropine 0.4 mg/mL for bradycardia, adenosine 3 mg/mL for SVT, amiodarone 50 mg/mL for arrhythmias. These concentrations provide appropriate volumes for pediatric weight-based dosing.

Case Example: Concentration Selection for Clinical Safety

Maria Santos, a 65-year-old woman in septic shock, requires norepinephrine for blood pressure support. She weighs 70 kg and needs an initial dose of 0.1 mcg/kg/min with titration capability.

Concentration selection: Standard norepinephrine 8 mg in 250 mL (32 mcg/mL) provides appropriate concentration for this patient. Alternative 4 mg in 250 mL (16 mcg/mL) would require higher infusion rates for equivalent doses.

Initial calculation: 0.1 mcg/kg/min × 70 kg × 60 min/hr ÷ 32 mcg/mL = 13.1 mL/hr initial rate. This rate allows precise titration in small increments while providing adequate duration before bag changes.

Titration planning: Protocol allows increases of 0.05 mcg/kg/min every 5 minutes. This equals 6.6 mL/hr increment (0.05 × 70 × 60 ÷ 32), providing precise titration capability within pump programming limits.

Equipment Specifications and Limitations

Infusion Pump Capabilities

Modern infusion pumps provide sophisticated delivery control with built-in safety features, but understanding their capabilities and limitations ensures safe, effective medication administration. Pump specifications affect calculation approaches and administration planning.

Flow rate ranges vary by pump model but typically deliver 0.1-999 mL/hr for most general-purpose pumps. Syringe pumps usually deliver 0.1-99 mL/hr with higher precision for small volumes. Some critical care pumps support rates up to 1,500 mL/hr for fluid resuscitation scenarios.

Programming precision affects calculation rounding decisions. Most pumps accept tenths of mL/hr (26.7 mL/hr), while some critical care models accept hundredths (26.75 mL/hr). Match your calculation precision to pump capabilities to avoid programming errors.

Volume limitations depend on pump design and intended use. General infusion pumps typically accommodate 50 mL to 3,000 mL containers. Syringe pumps usually accept 10 mL to 60 mL syringes. Large-volume pumps for blood products and fluid resuscitation may handle up to 5,000 mL containers.

Smart pump drug libraries provide additional safety features by checking programmed doses against established parameters. These systems calculate doses automatically when you input patient weight and desired dose, but you must verify that smart pump calculations match your manual calculations.

Syringe Selection Guidelines

Proper syringe selection affects measurement accuracy and administration safety. Choose syringe sizes appropriate for calculated volumes while considering precision requirements and administration routes.

Volume-to-syringe matching guidelines recommend using syringes that accommodate calculated volumes in the middle 50% of syringe capacity for optimal accuracy. For 0.5 mL medication, use 1 mL syringe. For 2.5 mL medication, use 3 mL or 5 mL syringe.

Precision considerations vary by syringe size and graduation markings. 1 mL syringes typically graduate in 0.01 mL increments, providing excellent precision for small volumes. 3 mL syringes graduate in 0.1 mL increments, suitable for moderate volumes. Larger syringes sacrifice precision for volume capacity.

Route-specific syringe requirements affect selection decisions. IV push medications often use 1-3 mL syringes for precise control. IM injections typically use 1-3 mL syringes with appropriate needle lengths. Subcutaneous injections usually employ 1 mL syringes or insulin syringes for small volumes.

IV Access Gauge Limitations

IV catheter gauge affects infusion capabilities and medication compatibility. Understanding gauge limitations helps plan administration strategies and prevents complications from inappropriate access choices.

Flow rate capabilities decrease with smaller gauge catheters. 14-gauge catheters support rapid fluid infusion up to 300 mL/min. 18-gauge catheters allow moderate flow rates up to 100 mL/min. 22-gauge catheters limit flow to approximately 35 mL/min. 24-gauge catheters restrict flow to 15-20 mL/min maximum.

Medication compatibility considerations include viscosity and pH factors. Blood products require 18-gauge or larger catheters to prevent hemolysis. Vesicant chemotherapy often needs central access to prevent tissue damage. High-concentration medications may require dilution for peripheral administration.

Case Example: Equipment Selection for Optimal Outcomes

Jennifer Martinez, a 45-year-old woman with pneumonia, needs vancomycin 1.5 g IV over 90 minutes. She has a 20-gauge peripheral IV in her left forearm.

Volume calculation: Vancomycin 1.5 g mixed in 250 mL normal saline per pharmacy protocol. Infusion rate = 250 mL ÷ 1.5 hours = 167 mL/hr.

Equipment assessment: 20-gauge IV catheter supports 167 mL/hr infusion rate adequately. General infusion pump can deliver this rate with appropriate precision. No equipment limitations prevent safe administration.

Administration planning: Program pump for 167 mL/hr over 1.5 hours. Monitor IV site closely during infusion for signs of infiltration or phlebitis. Vancomycin's potential for causing phlebitis requires careful IV site assessment.

Safety Protocol Checklists

High-Alert Medication Verification Procedures

High-alert medications require systematic verification procedures that go beyond routine calculation checking. These protocols provide multiple safety barriers to prevent errors that could cause severe patient harm.

Independent calculation verification requires two qualified staff members to perform calculations separately, then compare results before administration. Both practitioners must document their calculations and verify agreement before proceeding. Disagreements require resolution through pharmacy consultation or supervisor involvement.

Concentration verification procedures include checking medication labels against calculation assumptions, verifying expiration dates and storage requirements, and confirming that selected concentrations match calculation parameters. Many institutions use barcode scanning to verify medication identity before administration.

Patient identification verification becomes especially critical with high-alert medications because errors can cause rapid, severe harm. Use at least two patient identifiers (name, date of birth, medical record number) and match them against medication orders and administration records.

Route verification protocols ensure medications are given by intended routes, preventing dangerous route errors that can cause severe complications. Verify that calculated doses and volumes are appropriate for the intended administration route and patient condition.

Pre-Administration Safety Checks

Systematic pre-administration checks catch errors before they reach patients, providing the final safety barrier in medication administration. These checks should become automatic habits that you perform consistently regardless of time pressure or distractions.

"Five Rights" verification includes right patient, right medication, right dose, right route, and right time. Many institutions add additional rights: right documentation, right reason, right response. Verify each element systematically before every medication administration.

Dose reasonableness assessment involves evaluating calculated doses for clinical appropriateness. Does the calculated dose fall within expected ranges for the patient's condition, age, and weight? Unusual doses warrant verification before administration.

Patient assessment correlation ensures that calculated medications match current patient conditions and needs. Has the patient's clinical status changed since the medication was ordered? Do current vital signs and symptoms support medication administration?

Case Example: Safety Protocol Application

Michael Thompson, a 72-year-old man with atrial fibrillation, needs digoxin 0.25 mg IV. His calculated dose is 0.25 mg based on his age, weight, and kidney function.

High-alert verification process: Two nurses calculate independently— Nurse 1: Patient weight 75 kg, loading dose 10 mcg/kg = 750 mcg = 0.75 mg total, divided over 24 hours = approximately 0.25 mg IV now. Nurse 2: Uses different approach—

patient age >65, creatinine normal, standard initial dose 0.25 mg IV per protocol ✓

Pre-administration checks: Right patient (verify ID band and verbal confirmation), right medication (digoxin), right dose (0.25 mg), right route (IV), right time (as ordered). Patient assessment shows heart rate 95 bpm irregular, appropriate for digoxin administration.

Documentation: Both nurses sign verification documentation. Administer medication slowly IV push over 2-3 minutes. Monitor heart rate and rhythm closely for therapeutic response and toxicity signs.

Clinical Integration: Connecting Calculations with Care

These clinical correlation tables bridge the gap between mathematical accuracy and safe patient care by providing the contextual information needed for informed clinical decision-making. Understanding how calculations fit within specialty-specific protocols, equipment limitations, and safety procedures distinguishes competent practitioners from those who perform calculations mechanically.

Your ability to integrate calculation skills with clinical knowledge enables you to make appropriate decisions about medication preparation, administration routes, and safety protocols while maintaining the accuracy standards that protect patient safety. These correlations become intuitive through clinical experience and deliberate practice with realistic scenarios.

The safety protocols and verification procedures outlined here provide systematic approaches to error prevention that work reliably under pressure and time constraints. Consistent application of these protocols creates safety habits that protect both patients and practitioners throughout your career.

Key Takeaways for Clinical Correlation

- Specialty-specific calculation requirements reflect unique patient populations and acuity levels that demand adapted approaches
- Standard medication concentrations reduce calculation complexity while maintaining safety through consistency and predictability
- Equipment specifications and limitations affect calculation approaches and require consideration during administration planning
- Safety protocol checklists provide systematic verification procedures that prevent errors before they reach patients
- Clinical correlation knowledge distinguishes competent practitioners who integrate mathematical skills with clinical judgment effectively

References

1. Adams, M. P., Holland, L. N., & Urban, C. (2023). *Pharmacology for nurses: A pathophysiologic approach* (7th ed.). Pearson Education.
2. Agency for Healthcare Research and Quality. (2019). Medication reconciliation. *Patient Safety Network.* https://psnet.ahrq.gov/primer/medication-reconciliation
3. American Nurses Association. (2021). *Nursing: Scope and standards of practice* (4th ed.). ANA Publishing.
4. Brown, M., & Mulholland, J. (2024). *Drug calculations: Ratio and proportion problems for clinical practice* (12th ed.). Elsevier.
5. Clayton, B. D., Willihnganz, M. J., & Kimble, L. P. (2023). *Clayton's basic pharmacology for nurses* (19th ed.). Elsevier.
6. Institute for Safe Medication Practices. (2022). *ISMP's list of high-alert medications in acute care settings.* https://www.ismp.org/recommendations/high-alert-medications-acute-list
7. Karch, A. M. (2023). *Focus on nursing pharmacology* (9th ed.). Wolters Kluwer.
8. Morris, D. G. (2022). *Calculate with confidence* (8th ed.). Elsevier.
9. National Council of State Boards of Nursing. (2023). *NCLEX-RN examination: Test plan for the National Council Licensure Examination for Registered Nurses.* NCSBN.
10. Pickar, G. D., & Swart, B. (2023). *Dosage calculations* (11th ed.). Cengage Learning.
11. Potter, P. A., Perry, A. G., Stockert, P. A., & Hall, A. M. (2023). *Fundamentals of nursing* (11th ed.). Elsevier.
12. Richardson, M. (2024). *Drug calculations for nurses: A step-by-step approach* (6th ed.). McGraw-Hill Education.
13. Rosenthal, L. D., & Burchum, J. R. (2024). *Lehne's pharmacotherapeutics for advanced practice nurses and physician assistants* (3rd ed.). Elsevier.

14. The Joint Commission. (2023). *National Patient Safety Goals effective January 2023: Hospital accreditation program.* TJC Resources.
15. Thompson, J. M., McFarland, G. K., Hirsch, J. E., & Tucker, S. M. (2022). *Mosby's clinical nursing* (8th ed.). Elsevier.